T0326611

Resourcing Hope for Ageing and Dying in a Broken World

Resourcing Hope for Ageing and Dying in a Broken World

Wayfaring Through Despair

Ashley Moyse

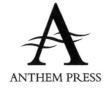

ANTHEM PRESS

Anthem Press
An imprint of Wimbledon Publishing Company
www.anthempress.com

This edition first published in UK and USA 2022
by ANTHEM PRESS
75–76 Blackfriars Road, London SE1 8HA, UK
or PO Box 9779, London SW19 7ZG, UK
and
244 Madison Ave #116, New York, NY 10016, USA

British Library Cataloguing-in-Publication Data
A catalogue record for this book is available from the British Library.

Library of Congress Cataloging-in-Publication Data
A catalog record for this book has been requested.

ISBN-13: 978-1-78527-861-7 (Hbk)
ISBN-10: 1-78527-861-4 (Hbk)

Cover credit: Cover image: By Eve Leader/Eveleader.com

This title is also available as an e-book.

To Grandma and Patricia. To Mom.

To those older persons of my past who have each shared their humanity with me, in the fulness of their corporeality, in their living and their dying, that I too might be humanised.

You feel you are hedged in; you dream of escape; but beware of mirages. Do not run or fly away in order to get free: rather dig in the narrow place which has been given you; you will find God there and everything. God does not float on your horizon, he sleeps in your substance. Vanity runs, love digs. If you fly away from yourself, your prison will run with you and will close in because of the wind of your flight; if you go deep down into yourself it will disappear in paradise.

—Gustave Thibon, quoted by Gabriel Marcel at the conclusion of a lecture delivered for the *Institute Supérieur de Pédagogie*, 13 December 1942.

(Gabriel Marcel, 'The Ego and Its Relationship to Others', in *Homo Viator: Introduction to the Metaphysics of Hope*, trans. Emma Craufurd and Paul Seton (South Bend: St Augustine's, 2010), 7–22 [22]).

CONTENTS

ACKNOWLEDGEMENTS

This book has emerged from experiences with others, ageing and dying, frail and finite. It has emerged from experiences of dialogue with these persons and through conversation with philosophers and theologians, living and dead. It has emerged with the memory of my mother and grandmother and others with whom, immersed in the fullness of living in time as our bodies, I have been gifted with such encounters through which I am learning to understand the human condition. And I am grateful.

Recognition must also go to the many persons with whom I have learned, discussed, argued, presented and published bits of this book along the way. These persons include Nigel Biggar, Farr Curlin, Chris Gilleard, Virginia Dunn, Sarah Harper, Ross Hastings, Joshua Hordern, Fabrice Jotterand, George Leeson, John C. McDowell, Seamus O'Mahony, Autumn Alcott Ridenour, David Robinson, Richard Topping, Héctor Velázquez, Els van Wijngaarden, Jens Zimmermann and a host of others. A special thanks must go to my friend and colleague Lydia S. Dugdale: that you read 'chapter four and everything else' with such care and have offered a thoughtful response to the book is cherished, truly. Thank you. To have such colleagues and friends who take interest in my work, offering both critique and praise, support and encouragement, is humbling, edifying and humanising.

Thanks also to my former students with whom I have had the honour of learning. These students have the courage to share their work with me, through which dynamic and engaging conversations have emerged. I am very proud of your accomplishments and grateful for all that you have taught me! Thanks especially to Victoria von der Leyen, Edward Chan Stroud, Maria Beer Vuco and Jessica Wyatt: You have each been instrumental in my thinking throughout the development of this particular project! And to David Bennet, Paul Charles, Paul Robinson and Ana Worthington, your research assistance, your collegiality, your good humour and our conversations are cherished—needed too!

To the team at Anthem Press, your patience with this project is appreciated. I want to thank, especially, Megan Grieving and Jabaslin Hephzibah as well as the reviewers who have served their roles well – offering both candour and encouragement, critique and constructive comment. Thank you. To those in the production team, managed by Sreejith Govindan, and to Paul Sutliff who helped to craft the index, I offer my sincere appreciation for your diligence and expertise.

That I have published three essays from which this volume has emerged also requires attention be given to the editors, reviewers, journals and/or presses that I've previously engaged and have received permission or licence to repurpose material – I am thankful.

Accordingly, this book includes material from the following:

(1) Ashley Moyse, "Fodder for Despair, Masquerading as Hope: Diagnosing the Postures of Hope(lessness) at the End of Life," *Religions*, vol. 10, no. 12 (2019): 651f. doi: 10.3390/rel10120651. This article is published under Creative Commons Attribution 4.0 International licence (CC BY 4.0) and is represented with modifications principally in chapter three, with content also found throughout this volume.

(2) Ashley John Moyse, "Bearing the Burdens we (don't Tend to) Bare," *Journal of Population Ageing*, vol. 13, no. 4 (September 2021): doi: 10.1007/s12062-021-09339-1. This article is published under Creative Commons Attribution 4.0 International licence (CC BY 4.0) and is represented with modifications principally in chapter two, with content also found throughout this volume.

(3) Ashley John Moyse (and trans. Maria Beer Vuco), "El significado actual del dolor y el sufrimiento en la era tecnológica," in *Sociedad Tecnológica y Futuro Humano, vol.2: El ser humano en la era tecnológica*, edited by H. Velázquez (Chile: Tirant Le Banch, 2021). A modified version of the original English essay is used, with permission, in the first chapter and throughout this volume.

I must also acknowledge funders who have supported my research or related conferences along the way. First, to the University of Divinity (Melbourne), where I was an honorary postdoctoral research fellow at Trinity College Theological School. The award received from UD helped to fund early research assistance (2017–2018), which contributed significantly to the genesis of this project and related outcomes. A Wellcome Trust Institutional Strategic Support Fund (ISSF) was received and used to facilitate the 2020 McDonald Centre Annual Conference at the University of Oxford ('Ageing and Despair: Towards Patience and Hope for Health and Care'). Thanks also to Peter,

Jonathan, Mark and others at the McDonald Agape Foundation (MAF). The continuing support and encouragement for the work being done through the McDonald Centre for Theology, Ethics and Public Life in the Faculty of Theology and Religion at the University of Oxford is sincerely valued.

Finally, for Aime and Theodore: Thank you for digging into those narrow spaces *with* me! 'I hope in Thee for us' (Gabriel Marcel).

Introduction

DIAGNOSING DESPAIR, RESOURCING HOPE

She was 75 when she died. My mother experienced a haemorrhagic stroke at the end of the first week of March 2020. It was a medical emergency none of us had expected given that Mom was generally healthy, vibrant and strong. She was an icon of 'successful ageing'.

At 75, that early Saturday morning, my mother awoke otherwise well, save for the persistent aches in her feet, knees and back that had become commonplace signs of her corporeality – discomforts and pains earned through her 45-year career, giving of herself for the care of others as a Registered Nurse (a vocation from which she had only recently retired). Moments later that same morning, calling out to my father that she could not see and that something was wrong, he corrected her stumbling about and laid her upon the nearby sofa. She exclaimed, 'I'm scared!' – and she said little else thereafter. Her healthful state was catastrophically altered in a moment. Her death followed eight days later. At 75, robust and active, my mother's death was unexpected – thwarting plans she and my father had made for their next several years together. At 75, my mother died.

Ezekiel Emanuel has written that he *wants* to die at 75.[1] Seventy-five, according to Emanuel, is an ideal age to die – living too long thereafter becomes a mere record of losses. Such losses include, for Emanuel, diminished productivity and other functions of one's work–life or industrious leisure. The life experienced following such changes, forced onto persons by age-related losses, is, as Emanuel suggests, *meaningless*. His desire is to avoid such cases of old age – and he challenges anyone who might suggest otherwise.[2] Escape from such a life is his answer to the problem of old age.

While Emanuel is not likely to pursue assisted dying, or suicide by his own hand,[3] Emanuel posits the depredations of ageing to become insufferable the longer persons live – suffering a life worse than death. A provocative claim that others might echo. But Emanuel has written without the experience of being 75 or any older than that. He is certainly, like all reading this sentence, ignorant of death too. Although I can imagine, as an oncologist he might argue otherwise, repeating, perhaps, as such: 'Doctors—those pragmatists who have seen death and stepped in to stop it, or at least to delay it, or to make it easier—*know* death and can do something about it.'[4] And perhaps that is where our critical examination of such 'knowledge' might begin. 'Knowing' of losses incurred in later life and knowing of how to die, yet alienated from the experiences of both, Emanuel offers his reader an imperative, which he considers right not only for his case but also for all other cases of later life where an accounting of losses mounts: actions that enable life with losses – after 75 – ought not to be deployed. That is to say, medical care beyond a particular calculus of chronometric age and losses seems 'counterproductive' – simply prolonging the cases of unwanted life.[5]

I would, however, challenge Emanuel. Sure, doctors do know much. This is true – incontestably. They are expert to know well the mechanisms that regulate bodily functions and can, with skill, mitigate many deleterious aberrations in such functions through pharmacological, surgical and technological intervention. Often observing the human body 'as a machine, as dead matter in motion', physicians and surgeons deploy their knowledge and demonstrate power over the body – any body.[6] Thus, for such physicians, a sick or frail or dying body is as any other, a case where expert knowledge can be exercised – extending or ending life accordingly. However, as some might suggest, doctors do not grapple with the depredations of ageing and dying in any meaningful way – with 'humility', as Gillian Rose claimed, while dying.[7] The confidence of knowledge can obscure openness to such meaning.

That is to say, while reading Emanuel, for example, one does get a sense of a meaningful life. Contra humility, however, it is meaning with certainty. Meaning is correlated with a case of life lived with robust capacities and productive functions. It is the meaningful life of the well-working machine – until it isn't. The body, *any* body, it seems, is as 'a heart-pumping, breath-gasping body [...] a material fleshy casing that is alien to him in many ways—the strangest and most repugnant way being that it aches and bleeds and will decay and die'.[8] Emanuel, thus, prognosticates with an expert's knowledgeable perspective but remains, it seems, *unavailable*[9] to reflect differently about particular experiences and meaning of later life – both his own and others. Instead, 'the hardening categories' of productivity and loss have seemingly ordered a valuation of meaning that remains closed off to new possibilities.[10] He has accepted, by the cases, an imperative for himself and others, relative to the problems of health or sickness. And by such acceptance, Emanuel might have closed himself off to encounter meaning differently; remaining 'not only occupied but encumbered with [his] own self'.[11] Allow me to explain, beginning with a brief discussion about the complex experiences of health and illness each person must live at every moment, at every age.

Regarding health and illness, I think it important to emphasise the 'and' in that phrase. Although, having previously trained in applied physiology, I used to teach otherwise in my early years of lecturing for a faculty of health sciences. At least I did teach as such until I started to read Friedrich Nietzsche and Karl Barth, for example, while retraining in theology.

Considering the former, after reading a brief aphorism in Nietzsche's *The Will to Power*, I began to question the binary poles and my preoccupations with measurement and classification, I had previously explained to students, drawing upon the biostatistical model of health and both the 1948 WHO definition, which posits health negatively (as the absence of disease or infirmity), but also positively with an exacting, maximal, depiction of (*complete* physical, mental and social) well-being as well as the functioning classifications offered by the WHO International Classification of Functioning, Disability and Health[12]: 'Health and sickness are not essentially different, as the ancient physicians and some practitioners even today suppose. One must not make of them distinct principles or entities that fight over the living organism and turn it into their arena.'[13] Consequently curious of the way I had conceived health previously, I turned towards the study of various philosophies of health.[14]

And through reflection and experience, I've come to realise differently. Understanding accordingly, that health and sickness are not particular and discrete phenomena, while also learning from the latter, vis-á-vis Barth, I began to perceive health in new light. Understanding the experience of health and illness, I recognised that we all live, together, 'the healthy and sick life of [our] soul and body and *with the life* of [our] body'.[15] So recognising and living as such (increasingly aware of the particularities of corporeality, my own and others), health and sickness is not adequately delimited by mean and measure. Although, such abstractions do provide helpful details which require both attention and, often, actionable response, but such details of knowledge ought not to be mistaken for understanding. Understanding is a mystery.

What is meant by 'mystery'? To be sure, it does not mean that one rejects the objective evidence of health and illness, which one might acquire through deductive study gained through physical medicine (a doctor's learned observation of your body as one of many bodies she observes – and has observed comparatively) and the data acquired through more invasive means of analysis. But mystery refuses to attend to the reality of the healthy and sick life of bodies, in all of their complex particularity, as mere cases where sympathies are expressed but, 'when all is said and done, I am obliged to admit that I feel absolutely nothing'.[16] Rather, the meaning of mystery, in this instance, is informed by the writings of Gabriel Marcel whose influence and thinking will feature (although not solely) throughout this book: with the healthy *and* sick life of our body, we are immersed in the events of human existence.

Such immersion means that we participate necessarily in the mystery of being – 'a sphere where the distinction between what is in me and what is before me loses its meaning and its validity'.[17] Jan Baars explains such immersive experience, suggesting '"mystery" refers to some "thing" that I cannot place in front of me to get a clear look at it because I am always already *involved* in it and *preoccupied* with it'[18] – it is 'something in which I find myself caught up'.[19] Thus, immersed, involved, preoccupied and caught up, the '*mystery of our being* involves the active situation that we are concerned with—our experience—and so, is one whose true nature can only be grasped, acknowledged, or recognized from the inside'.[20] And 'from the inside', Marcel regards the recuperative act of reflection (a dialectic moving back and forth between experience and thought), which contemplates the realities of bodily experience, the realities of being a body, as principal for understanding.

Experiencing the mystery of being, thus pursuing that question 'Am I am my life?'[21] in the healthy and sick life of our body, we thus differentiate being (mystery) a body from having (problem) a body. The difference is not insignificant.

For Marcel, 'a problem is something that lies more or less objectively before me to be solved, such as an engine that does not function'.[22] The problematic body is the abstracted body, it is as the *every* or *universal* body, which remains as fodder for pure, dispassionate observation. The states of healthfulness *or* illness, states delimited by function or dysfunction relative to the abstracted standard body, are reduced to a mere quandary or artefact we can represent or possess by the numbers or working parts, and which can be exhausted, surveyed and managed by particular techniques. It is in this way that Marcel regards 'A problem [as] something met', as a thing 'which bars my passage. It is before me in its entirety'.[23]

Marcel admits the world of problems is valuable and the knowledge gained is often good (we would be naïve to cast aside, uncritically, the many goods produced by such knowledge); but the world of mystery is ontologically grounding – it is of a higher good.[24] For clarity, 'one might say that the human person encounters both problems and mysteries and must investigate each accordingly'.[25] As a higher good, however, 'one must resist the temptation of reducing the mysteries of life into problems'.[26] Yet the circumstances of the human condition can upset the ranking order. These circumstances 'depend upon the social and cultural conditions into which we have been socialized'.[27] These circumstances reflect, one might argue, the social imaginaries incumbent to a particular society, not only through but also within which persons and societies repeat associated practices that might legitimise the social imaginary.[28] Hartmut Rosa contends, of the circumstances of our modern situatedness, 'We learn and become habituated to a certain practical attitude toward the world'.[29] For Rosa, the practical attitude, or modern social imaginary (and related practices), is *aggressive* – 'Everything that appears to us must be known, mastered, conquered, made useful'.[30] Such learning and habituation, concomitantly for Marcel, educates us to see everything as a problem. As such, the world of problems over-prioritised can occlude the existential reflection and higher order of understanding (mystery); it can advantage the objective study of and knowledge over *things*; and it can excite (or train) universalising and functionalising perspectives (habits) that degrade human life.[31] (And many of us have already been trained to prioritise such perspective: 'we are forced to admit that the more techniques advance, the more reflection is thrust into the background'. Moreover, 'what does seem certain is that the progress and above all the extreme diffusion of techniques tends to create a spiritual and intellectual atmosphere [or more precisely, an anti-spiritual and anti-intellectual atmosphere] as unfavourable as possible to the exercise of reflection'.)[32]

Frailty in later life and the fact of disease, both pain and suffering, can furnish such a circumstance, in which we forget of mystery, of 'being-in-a-situation' which cannot be adequately explained from 'any high terrace' of abstraction.[33] Yet habits of the problematic life, which can excite such forgetfulness, do blur our reflections on mystery and invigorate the study of problems for persons living through the healthy and sick lives of their body. Such facts of frailty and disease, after all, encroach upon and challenge our experiences of the life of our bodies while they impair or weaken our strength to live. Even that event where we have stubbed our toe upon the footing of furniture in the dark of night and think all calamity has befallen us can weaken our strength to live – at very least, I admit, I have found myself exclaiming, alongside particular expletives, 'Oh, God, take me now!'

For many, maybe most all, such encroachments and challenges excite an existential anxiety; for some, a destabilizing dialectic of fear and desire is provoked. That we do grow old and frail, that we are susceptible to injury and illness, is but a reminder, after all, that with the healthy and sick life of our body death is certain. We know of our mortality. Such knowledge is unsettling.

That we will grow old and die is the ground or the nature of our anxiety: 'the agony of a creature living in time, the agony of feeling one's-self at the mercy of time'.[34] Or, as Ernest Becker has written, highlighting the anxiety of finitude, 'It is a terrifying dilemma to be in and to have to live with [...] But to live a whole lifetime with the fate of death haunting one's dreams and even the most sun-filled days—that's something else'.[35] Immersed as we are in *this* time-bound life, in the healthy and sick life of our bodies, our anxiety, that agony of our existence, can goad relentlessly both desires and fears – both of which are 'bound up with expectation'.[36] (And as Becker posits, we erect a range of death-denying narratives and practices through which we might gain escape from such angst[37]).

So provoked, such anxiety can reduce our perspective from whence we see life, bound by time and fated by finitude, as a problem, which we do not desire (which we do not deserve).[38] As a problem, the body loses its grounding, that is , its existential normativity, while the abstractions of ideals of form and function take precedence.

Desire and fear are accompanied then, rather preceded, by an enclosing perception that our life is as (or ought be considered like) any other problem, which one can analyse and resolve by way of overt rational (whether industrial, digital, political or moral) technique.[39] Our life becomes like sheets of heavy-bond paper we have in our possession and that we wish to shape to ideal form; and scissors are all that we need to cut to order the facts of our life, these sheets of paper.[40] For Marcel, this is indicative of the problematic life – or the broken perspective of the problematic individual, who 'treats every encounter, person, or thing [including the self] [...] as a fact, because facts can be categorized, systematized, and [ultimately] solved'.[41]

Our life, as a problematic case, becomes reduced to a compendium of constituent parts, possessions we *have* to manage life rather than the metaphysical *being* we are that lives life. Rather, 'When man begins to become a problem to himself, the problematic man defines the self either by possessions he has or the profession he engages in. [...] By raising objects to the level of what is existentially meaningful, the problematic man can classify, systematize, order, and so, he believes—exert control over what constitutes his identity'.[42] The broken perspective is a quagmire within which we build a 'broken world'.[43] It is a world broken by an imaginary and the corresponding complex processes of socialisation that favours *control over* rather than *life in* the world – where science is enabled to expand knowledge, where technology manages the world disclosed by science, where economic development conflates control with consumption (of knowledge and instrument) and where legal and political schema ensure the social preconditions and processes through which we become habituated can be anticipated and organised.[44] The broken perspective constructs a broken world where everything is reduced to a mere problem.

It is within such worlds that we simply *have* life. Possessing life as such, the problems identified, perceived through desires and fears, are thought as those which can and ought to be fixed. Fixing the world, which we have, corresponds to the setting of *things* to order – an order that suits our desires, or amends our fears. It is a world constructed upon an idealised feedback loop. Responding positively to desires (enhancing) and negatively to fears (reducing) thus becomes the principal aim of the problematic life. And ethics becomes a mere function of calculus. For Marcel, among others critical of the current age, this principal aim is the fundamental position taken on by those conformed to the 'broken world', a world pedagogically nurtured by the social practices incumbent to (late) modern imaginings[45] and situated by complementary but flattened moral utility and abstracted imperatives.

'Having' life in this sense, in this broken world, is concerned with *possessing* the discrete functions of one's living (both 'vital and social'[46]), which can be gained or lost, produced or perished: 'We are tempted to think that no longer having anything is the same as no longer being anything: and in fact, the general trend [...] is to identify one's-self with what one has'[47] – whether one has youthfulness, healthfulness, self-determination, independence, choice, control and the like. Such a life, as above, is one 'given over to desire and fear'.[48] Marcel thus laments: the individual, having learned to see herself (and with everyone else) as a constellation of functional (or functionalizing) *things*, is coerced by such thinking to seek out, to secure and to protect such functions. Her hope resides with such capacities and commodities. Thus, the response to dysfunction(ing) becomes increasingly predictable and patterned, viz. homogenised. Herbert Marcuse would describe such an individual and others like her, and the society within which such individuals stand, as *one-dimensional* – disciplined by the instrumental reasoning that problems habituate.[49]

Of course, desires and fears are but designations we assign to the problems of functioning *things* we wish that we might gain or keep and dread that we might (or do) lose. Technological solutions are, thus, presented as interventions to ensure we might secure desires or remove fears: 'fear (along with desire) is at the heart of the problematic, as every technique is at the service of some fear (or desire)'.[50] And it is the problematic that corresponds most presciently in our forthcoming discussions concerning ageing and dying, because fear and desire, as Marcel so understands, corresponds to losses (whether present experiences or future forfeitures) of 'things' that we see ourselves 'possessing'.[51]

Corresponding to such discussions are those institutions and programmes, policies and professionals, which too have been schooled by the 'characteristic feature of our age'[52]; in other words, that persistent ideal that 'everything can be explained exhaustively',[53] and either enhanced or fixed. Schooled in such a way that a prevailing attitude persists: we needn't to be available for others (in the world) intimately, with a novel presence,[54] but can manage others (and their problems) as we managed ourselves productively by resolving and ultimately controlling both vital and social functions through repetitions of technological intervention. Such schooling teaches us that individuals' problems, like any other problems, can and should 'be overhauled' when such harms of 'disorderly elements – sickness, accidents of every sort – will break in on the smooth working' of the life we *have*.[55]

Perhaps, as a physician, Emanuel knows too well that the doctor's 'inspection bench' and hospital 'repair shop' cannot, in the end, resolve the problem of desires and assuage the problem of fears, when persons confront the inevitability of corporeality, which includes later life, disease, decay and death. As Seamus O'Mahony laments, physicians, after all, might be 'treating, and over-treating' but they are 'not healing' persons living longer, persons baring the *problems* of corporeality that emerge as time grows heavy in them, proving the limits of technique and human life as finite.[56] Perhaps Emanuel's stance relative to the age of 75 reveals that he knows the riddle, which is the problem of life, cannot be resolved – he can offer neither 'security' nor 'guarantee' that one can fix the functions we *have* to live; refusing a different ground from which to apprehend life, he thus despairs.[57] Or, as Marcel comments,

> The world of the problematical is the world of fear and desire, which are inseparable; at the same time, it is the world of the functional—or of what can be functionalized [...]. Every technique serves, or can be made to serve, some desire or some fear; conversely, every desire as every fear tends to invent its appropriate technique. From this standpoint, despair consists in the recognition of the ultimate inefficacy of all technics, joined to the inability or the refusal to change over to a new ground—a ground where all technics are seen to be incompatible with the fundamental nature of being, which itself escapes our grasp.[58]

Perhaps it is that Emanual is asking this question and despairing the necessary answer: 'What can man achieve? [...] He can achieve as much as his technics; yet we are obliged to admit that these technics are unable *to save man himself*'.[59] I say 'despairingly' here because despair and desire (and fear) correspond. Despair, after all, is the result of 'frustrated desire, because with the loss of the thing desired, nothing else appears worthwhile or meaningful'.[60]

Of course, these introductory reflections on Emanuel's desperation that he *hopes* for death at the age of 75 might be regarded as mere conjecture. Although, I think they are diagnostic. Nevertheless here, in this introduction, these reflections raise a range of important concepts, explicitly and implicitly, which do persist throughout this book – abstracted objectivity and immersive existence, to have and to be, problem and mystery, desire (fear) and hope. These are concepts central to the writings of Marcel,[61] whose works have inspired my thinking and have centred my study of despair for persons who are growing older, confronting frailties and struggling to live while dying from disease and depredation. These are concepts essential for us to resource or recuperate hope for ageing and dying in a later modern world.

After all, for persons confronting existential anxieties, hope is needed.

But we must not be ignorant of differing modes and meanings of hope either – not all hopes can sustain us in times of calamity and crisis. Some hopes, as alluded to already above, offer concrete aims that are fodder for despair, risking life's end.[62] Other hopes torment, engendering a sort of longsuffering that never finds respite.[63] One must learn, therefore, to discern such risk, so as not to be perturbed by such hopes that are as the other evils contained in Pandora's *pithos* [jar].[64] One must learn to discover the fodder for despair, which introduces illusions (or dis-incarnate rationalist ideals[65]) of human being that do not attend to the actualities of corporeality or that masquerade as hope – functionalist hoping that only returns towards despair even while offering emancipatory flight from it. Such discovery might offer those persons confronting the actualities of frailty and decay, of ageing and dying, and vulnerable to the gravity of despair, a way to be(come) opened to recognise hope differently.

That some forms of hope are hopeless, is of primary concern. That despair can and does masquerade as hope, including for persons confronting the necessity and immanence of death, needs to be illumined. Discriminating or diagnosing despair and hope is the task of this book, while frailties in later life and irremediable diagnoses provide the content and contours from which we might gain understanding of the ethical life.

It is certainly true; hope is needed for those situations of 'struggle in the claws of death'.[66] Hope is needed where the depredations of aging reveal the finitude and frailty of the human condition. Hope is needed also for those confronting the limits of human life antagonised by the forerunners of death, whether decay or disease. Hope is needed for those of us storied by late modern imaginaries, imaginaries steeped in desire and wrought from the problematical, which shape the way we see ourselves and others, ageing and dying.

So shaped, persons prioritise desires for independence, autonomy, control and the like, which reveal prevailing attitudes about human being, frailty, ageing and death. Such priorities and attitudes are those that are habituated and thus have become familiar in our late modern age, which is also disciplined by the coinhering rationalities where market metaphors, technological imperatives and consequentialist analyses not only nurture but also are nurtured by our desires and fears that result in or risk despair. Accordingly, the following labours to diagnose the state of ageing and dying in our late modern age as one vulnerable to despair, without the resources to strengthen persons confronting existential anxieties. Thus, turning towards the mystery of 'being-in-a-situation' and the irreducible actualities of corporeality and community, of one's body and other bodies, I also introduce us afresh to the practices of being, of virtues, that might ready each of us, together, to live the healthy and sick life of our body-and-soul, to journey as wanderers, itinerant beings, towards later life and death, differently.

Hopefully.

* * * * *

Before reading further, I think of this book as a digest of sorts – illuminating reflections on later life and preoccupations in the 'broken world' of our late modern age. As a digest, I don't intend for this book, therefore, to offer a comprehensive and systematic examination of ageing and dying or the biopolitics that position and coerce bodies in public settings like hospitals, hospices, aged-care centres and the like. It is not an extensive examination of despair and hope, either. It is certainly not an exegetical analysis of Marcel's philosophy or Ivan Illich's *Medical Nemesis*, or Dietrich Bonhoeffer's understanding of vicarious representative action, as you will see.

It is, however, a witness. That is to say, with this book I have taken up the task to bear witness to the *broken world*, where objective, functionalising and dispassionate powers of primary reflection are overprioritised.[67] Thus, what follows is not merely a parsing and organization of relevant text and argument, traversing disciplines, so that a reader can walk away with further epistemic resources to be used or discarded as though knowledge stands in reserve. Although there is such work within the following pages. Bearing witness, the following reflects upon experiences of frailty in later life and irremediable disease (foregrounding experiences of ageing and dying and the anxieties of corporeality), while illuminating the brokenness of the world I see and sense through such reflections. Seeing and sensing of such fragmenting within persons despairing of their (and others') lives, I set a critical mood while searching conviction and a summoning call chart the creative, hopeful response. The book has thus developed like a cartographer's map, which charts the journey of life and contemplation as one wanders 'but with direction'.[68] That is to say, this book, encouraged by the writings of Marcel, includes several accounts of people and of corporeality, which permit the critical reflections and responses, oscillating back and forth between experience and reflection.

By way of reason and reflection, the following discerns a vulnerability to despair, experienced by ageing and dying persons (among others) – at very least among a constellation of persons ageing and dying in the modern, affluent West. The following considers the kind of hope which conceals despair for such persons hurtling towards death, feeling of life's old age, haunted by the depredations of frailty and caught up in the throes of terminal diagnoses and futile medical interventions. My critical reflections consider experiences of ageing and dying, as well as pain and suffering, in order to diagnose despair, which is concealed by a corrupted form of hope cultivated by late modern narratives that prioritise a series of coinhering ideals (i.e. technological rationalities [control over *things*], independence and self-determination). These ideals, among others, feature prominently in late modern narratives that consider pain and suffering, as well as corporeality and finitude, as problems to resolve by way of human agency – and the confluence of desire, rationalism and technique.

Accordingly, Chapter 1 introduces our study that moves, in the first instance, towards a diagnostic of despair experienced by ageing and dying persons, while attempting to understand the technological influence, or ontology, which has contributed to shaping the contours and content of a late modern imagination that prioritises particular ideals or ways of being and doing in the world. A critical study of technological imaginaries that have influenced the way persons not only say but also see the world, including themselves in (or against) it, anchors the analysis and the understanding of why it might be that the stories we tell ourselves have influenced why and how and where despair might haunt our existence. The following chapters show that such an understanding risks leaving persons either isolated from others or deceived by a pernicious hoping while ensnared by a persistent passion and without the habits that might resource a strength to flourish as human being, even unto death. Such despair disciplines persons towards a pessimistic preoccupation with both life and death while anticipating suicide or other, often tragic, outcomes that impede or greatly curtail or even completely inhibit human flourishing.

Chapter 2 studies the experiences of ageing – specifically, it aims to examine Fourth-age experiences marked by depredations, frailties and losses while critically interrogating Third-age preoccupations. The Fourth age is studied as the burden of older life, which exaggerate feelings of fear and desire while resourcing despair. However, while some such burdens are borne from human corporeality, others are socially constructed and afflict older persons further.

Consequently, Chapter 2 introduces a typology of burdens, identifying reflexive, transitive and accusative burdens. The reflexive dirge of the person grieving their losses of competence, self-sufficiency and independence includes a transitive counterpart, where a person's self-perceived burden also includes the sense that one has become a burden to others. The accusative burden is experienced when persons are marked by others, catastrophically, as a problem or encumbrance – a liability risking the upset of economics and social order, for example. These differing burdens must be given attention while attending to the ideations that prioritise independence but risk despair. Thus, the relation between burdened self-image, despair and late modern and policy preoccupations with independence further focuses such attention. Specifically, the prominence of independence in narratives of successful ageing are interrogated, as the chapter explores ageing, frailty and the existential distress of the oldest 'old' as well as those much younger but who fear becoming 'old'.

Turning our attention towards dying, Chapter 3 builds upon the previous while arguing that a late modern anthropology, cultivated by images of Heraclean self-sufficiency and self-determination, leaves persons vulnerable to despair but without the hope that can hasten patience to flourish as human beings while experiencing both the heights and depths of despair – a patience that permits human beings to flourish even unto death. Instead, that same anthropology entraps both persons and the medical institution, including the professionals formed within it, in a reciprocal chasing of individual, institutional, or professional agency (and technological rationality) in flight from, but hastening, ironically, further, despair.

Principally, the purpose is to demonstrate how late modern autonomy, or self-determining absolute agency, leaves persons at risk for despair. That same agency also determines not only negative dispositions concerning human limitations and functional losses (such limitations and losses are opposed to the ideal of the modern subject) but also the decisions for (voluntary or assisted) death. In fact, the risk for despair is occluded by the logic of a functional hoping and goaded by instrumental reasoning that makes voluntary (viz., controllability of) death essential for the modern subject. Put differently, Chapter 3, while studying the experiences and reasons of persons soliciting medical assistance in dying, illuminates the way 'hope' functions for many persons confronting the threats of death and the actualities of finitude. It shows that functional hoping is a 'hope' said to be conferred by autonomy. However, under further interrogation, functional hoping as a 'hope' is shown to be nothing but a temptation to despair in disguise.

Finally, seeking to think differently, hopefully, Chapter 4 reflects further on Marcel and the way of hope – examining his understanding of the human condition and the ethical life. With Marcel, as is evident already, we find a neighbour who is critical of the kind of imaginaries and flattened moral constructions that exaggerate existential anguish and offer no ground upon which persons might journey through despair. Moreover, with Marcel, 'we find an image of the human being that attends carefully to concrete experiences, that dwells on descriptions of personal experience, that values existence and tries not to ignore or lose it in concepts'.[69] He is a philosopher of existence who, as Julia Urabayen Pérez has described rightly, 'searches, questions, examines and walks while thinking or thinking while walking' through life's triumphs and tragedies.[70]

That Marcel draws upon his experiences and others, as well as the experiences of his characters portrayed in plays, for example, for the content of description and the concrete experience of human life is mirrored by my own experiences of ageing and dying – experiences shaped by my encounters with others. Such encounters have awakened an understanding that my fellows who stand before me claim me for responsibility – our own corporeal lives too, claim us; demanding that we respond to the exigencies of life. In neighbourly conversation, Chapter 4 also draws upon Dietrich Bonhoeffer's vision of responsibility as a complementary vision, which might shed more light upon moral realism and incarnate, intersubjective (thus loving) ethics that *are* ontologically hopeful.

The hopeful life is the responsible life. It is the intersubjective life. Both Marcel and Bonhoeffer set persons upon the ground upon which we are immersed in situations (of ageing and dying) and invited, as Gustave Thibon has suggested poetically in the epigraph, to 'dig in the narrow place which has been given'. The hopeful life as the responsible life is cultivated not by way of efficient technique that erect means for persons to fight against or to flee from the narrow place. Rather the hopeful life, as the responsible life, bears (inter)corporeal life and discovers strength, by the habits or practices of virtue, to understand the human condition. Yet it does not cling to life out of instrumental necessity either. Rather the hopeful life is a mystery within which all persons are caught up, alongside others, and understood through the experiences of and reflections on bodily life. Such understanding gifts persons with a perspective that enables the wayfarer's journey – allowing the struggle towards a reconciled future through the unclarities, calamities and catastrophes of a corporeal present where ageing and dying are real. Such hope digs, responsibly and lovingly, patiently and courageously, to live a human life, together, limited by frailty and finitude, delimited by the exceptions of each particular life (and the gathered community), in the midst of death.

Notes

1 Ezekiel J. Emanuel, 'Why I hope to die at 75', *The Atlantic* (October 2014). Accessed 20 January 2020 from https://www.theatlantic.com/magazine/archive/2014/10/why-i-hope-to-die-at-75/379329/.

2 Louise Aronson offers a thoughtful assessment of Emanuel's article and additional comments that raise question about meaning in later life (Louise Aronson, *Elderhood: Redefining Ageing, Transforming Medicine, Reimagining Life* (New York: Bloomsbury, 2021), 308–312). But her riposte to Emanuel's claim that later life becomes increasingly

meaningless as one is forced by depredations and disability to make accommodations for living, is particularly apropos. If the fact of 'adaptations were a problem', we ought then to lower the threshold age to 40 (Ibid., 310).

3 Louise Aronson reminds her readers, commenting on Emanuel's *wanting* to die at 75, that he has 'opposed euthanasia and physician-assisted suicide for decades' (Ibid., 308).

4 Jeffrey P. Bishop, *The Anticipatory Corpse: Medicine, Power, and the Care of the Dying* (Notre Dame: University of Notre Dame Press, 2011), 120. Emphasis is mine.

5 Aronson, *Elderhood*, 308.

6 Bishop, *Anticipatory Corpse*, 60.

7 Gillian Rose, *Love's Work: A Reckoning with Life* (New York: New York Review, 1995), 79.

8 Ernest Becker, *The Denial of Death* (New York: Free Press, 1973), 26.

9 Gabriel Marcel, 'On the Ontological Mystery', in *The Philosophy of Existence*, trans. Manya Harari (Providence: Cluny, 2018), 5–46 (40).

10 Ibid., 41.

11 Ibid., 42.

12 See the WHO's *Constitution* (Geneva: World Health Organization, 1948), https://www.who.int/about/governance/constitution and *International classification of functioning, disability and health* (Geneva: World Health Organization, 2001), https://www.who.int/standards/classifications/international-classification-of-functioning-disability-and-health. For further reflection on the WHO definition, see Jerome Bickenbach, 'WHO's Definition of Health: Philosophical Analysis', in *Handbook of the Philosophy of Medicine*, eds. Thomas Schramme and Steven Edwards (Dordrecht: Springer, 2017), 961–974.

13 Friedrich Nietzsche, *The Will to Power*, trans. Walter Kaufmann and Reginald J Hollingdale (New York: Vintage, 1968), 29.

14 Neil Messer's *Flourishing* offers an excellent and critically engaged summary of several of these philosophies offered by Christopher Boorse, Lennart Nordenfelt, Jerome Wakefield, S Kay Toombs and others, before turning to his constructive Barthian-Thomist theology of health. See Neil Messer, *Flourishing: Health, Disease, and Bioethics in Theological Perspective* (Grand Rapids: Eerdmans, 2013).

15 Karl Barth, *The Church Dogmatics*, trans. Geofrey Bromiley and Thomas Forsyth Torrance, 14-Volumes (Edinburgh: T&T Clark, 2004), III/4, 358. Emphasis is mine.

16 Marcel, 'Ontological Mystery', 40.

17 Gabriel Marcel, *Being and Having: An Existentialist Diary*, trans. Katherine Farrer (Westminster: Dacre, 1949), 117.

18 Jan Baars, *Aging and the Art of Living* (Baltimore: Johns Hopkins University Press, 2012), 184.

19 Marcel, *Being and Having*, 100.

20 Jill Graper Hernandez, *Gabriel Marcel's Ethics of Hope: Evil, God, and Virtue* (London: Bloomsbury, 2013), 13.

21 Marcel, *Being and Having*, 87.

22 Baars, *Aging and the Art of Living*, 184.

23 Marcel, *Being and Having*, 100.

24 Marián Palenčár, 'Gabriel Marcel and the question of human dignity', *Human Affairs* 27, no. 2 (2017): 116–130.

25 R. James Lisowski, 'Speaking of mystery: Evil and death in the philosophy of Gabriel Marcel and the resulting pastoral applications', *Marcel Studies* 4, no. 1 (2019): 13–24 (15).

26 Ibid., 15.

27 Hartmut Rosa, *The Uncontrollability of the World*, trans. James C. Wagner (Cambridge: Polity, 2021), 6

28 See Charles Taylor, *Modern Social Imaginaries* (Durham: Duke University Press, 2003); Charles Taylor, 'Modern social imaginaries', *Public Culture* 14, no. 1 (2002): 91–124; and Claudia Strauss, 'The imaginary', *Anthropological Theory* 6, no. 3 (2006): 322–344.

29 Rosa, *Uncontrollability of the World*, 6.

30 Ibid.

31 See Gabriel Marcel, *Man Against Mass Society*, trans. George S. Fraser (South Bend: St Augustine's, 2008).

32 Ibid., 7.

33 Gabriel Marcel, *The Mystery of Being, Volume I: Reflection and Mystery*, trans. George S. Fraser (South Bend: St Augustine's, 2001), 133.

34 Marcel, *Being and Having*, 73.

35 Becker, *Denial of Death*, 27.

36 Gabriel Marcel, *The Mystery of Being, Volume II: Faith and Reality* (South Bend: St Augustine's, 2001), 158.

37 On such escape, I recommend a very fine documentary film exploring Becker's thoughts, in conversation with Terror Management Theory experts and philosophers: Greg Bennick and Patrick Shen, *Flight from death: the quest for immortality* (A Documenary Film), narr. Gabriel Byrne (Arcadia: Transcendental Media, 2003).

38 Comparatively, Hartmut Rosa regards fear and anxiety as 'paradigmatic "resonance killers", as—at least when they are overpowering—they prevent the subject from opening it up to , tuning into, or becoming involved in the world. The subject tends to become *incapable of encounter*, even *immobilized*, as anxiety obstructs or impedes its ability to move *toward the world* [...]. In a state of anxiety [...] the subject is unavoidably concerned with *not being touched* and thus with avoiding potential resonances' (Hartmut Rosa, *Resonance: A Sociology of Our Relationship to the World*, trans. James C. Wagner (Cambridge: Polity, 2019), 121). Rosa continues, suggesting that desire, demeaned by objectivity, can also become as such, a resonance killer. And by resonance killer, Rosa means a way that closes off one's relating to and in and with the world, where persons (i.e., subjects) and world not only fail to meet but also remain inhibited to transform each other. Accordingly, resonance or world-relationship can be frustrated by fear, anxiety, and desire (even while these remain as basic elements for human subjectivity and relationship, which is not only bodily and reflexive but also cognitive and emotional) (Ibid., 110–124).

39 Marcel, *Being and Having*, 172.

40 Ashley John Moyse, *The Art of Living for the Technological Age: Toward a Humanizing Performance* (Minneapolist: Fortress, 2021), 23–34.

41 Hernandez, *Marcel's Ethics of Hope*, 5–9 (9).

42 Ibid., 6.

43 Marcel develops his idea of the broken world in his Gifford Lectures, delivered in Aberdeen, Scotland (1949 and 1950). In the first volume of these published lectures, 'Reflection and Mystery', Marcel remarks the broken world might be a world put in place, but it is a world that might not have a heart – having developed, for example, by the novel powers of modern science and technology, and the rationalist ordering of facts as knowledge, the possibility of 'self-destruction' or 'world-suicide'. The perspective is one rooted by the 'existence of a will to power' (Gabriel Marcel, *Mystery of Being* (I), 22). Within this essay, Marcel cites from his play *Le Monde cassé*, which you can read here: Gabriel Marcel, 'The Broken World: A Four Act Play',

in *Gabriel Marcel's Perspectives on the Broken World*, trans. Katharine R. Hanley (Milwaukee: Marquette University Press, 1998), 31–152.

44 Rosa, *Uncontrollability of the World*, 15–18.

45 While it is important to stress the plurality of modernities – there is not one way through which cultures have been modernised – Western modernity is, as Charles Taylor has argued, 'inseparable from a certain kind of social imaginary', which 'enables [...] the practices of [Western] society (Taylor, *Modern Social Imaginaries*, 1–2). As alluded already, with discussions from Taylor, Rosa, Marcel, and others, the following examines a range of 'new practices and institutional form (science, technology, [...]), of new ways of living (individualism, secularization, instrumental rationality); and of new forms of malaise (alienation, meaninglessness, [...])' (Ibid., 1), which give rise to the kind of over-prioritisation of the problematical that Marcel characterizes as 'broken'.

46 Marcel, 'Ontological Mystery', 6. Vital functions might be considered as those which are biological (i.e., physical and psychical) while social functions include those such as 'the consumer, the producer, the citizen, etc.' (7).

47 Marcel, *Being and Having*, 84.

48 Ibid., 76.

49 Herbert Marcuse, *One Dimensional Man: Studies in the Ideology of Advanced Industrial Society* (Boston: Beacon, 1991).

50 Jared Kemling, 'Anxiety and Fidelity: Gabriel Marcel on Existential Fear', *Kinesis* 40, no. 2 (2015): 75–83 (77).

51 Kemling, 'Anxiety and Fidelity', 79.

52 Marcel, 'Ontological Mystery', 6.

53 Rosa Slegers, 'Reflections on a Broken World: Gabriel Marcel and William James on Despair, Hope and Desire', in *Hope Against Hope: Philosophies, Cultures and Politics of Possibility and Doubt*, eds. Janet Horrigan and Ed Witse (Leiden: Brill, 2010), 55–74 (62).

54 Gabriel Marcel, *Creative Fidelity*, trans. Robert Rosthal (New York: Fordham University Press, 2002), 147–174.

55 Marcel, 'Ontological Mystery', 8.

56 Seamus O'Mahony, *Can Medicine Be Cured? The Corruption of a Profession* (London: Head of Zeus, 2019), 12. The imagery of the heaviness of time comes from Jean Améry, who presents time as that which accrues or accumulates within one's body, increasing its mass, making difficult the work of living in the world (See Jean Améry, *On Ageing: Resignation and Revolt*, trans. John D. Barlow (Indiana University Press, 1994), 1–26).

57 Marcel, 'Ontological Mystery', 25.

58 Ibid., 29.

59 Ibid., 29.

60 Slegers, 'Reflections on a Broken World', 56.

61 Not only central concepts but also coinhering concepts that work to reveal 'the human condition [...] [where] The second term in the pair expresses a more valuable and ontologically higher and better reality than the first' (Palenčár, 'Marcel and human dignity', 117.

62 Emil M. Cioran, *A Short History of Decay*, trans. Richard Howard (London: Penguin, 2018), 10–13, 143.

63 Friedreich Nietzsche, *Human, All Too Human: A Book for Free Spirits*, trans. Helen Zimmern (Edinburgh: T.N. Foulis), 82.

64 Pandora's *pithos* is first introduced by the Greek poet Hesiod, in his *Works and Days* (circa. 700 BCE). It follows the introduction of Prometheus who had tricked his god-fellows, including Zeus. Punishing humanity in response to Prometheus's trickery, Zeus conjures a plan to introduce evil to the world. Gifting the first woman, Pandora, to Epimetheus, Zeus enacted his plan. Epimetheus, the brother of Prometheus, was the caretaker of a jar which contained all the toils and sicknesses, among all other evils. But Pandora curiously opened the jar, releasing troubles and harms into the world, closing its seal just before hope, or 'deceptive expectations' was released (Franco Montanari, Chr. Tsagalis, and Antonios Rengakos, eds., *Brill's Companion to Hesiod* (Leiden: Brill, 2009), 77.)

65 One might find a corresponding sentiment in Charles Taylor's *A Secular Age* where he introduces a discussion of 'excarnate' life, which is incumbent to a modernity that elects to prefer forms of social and individual life that are rationalist rather than enfleshed. Briefly, excarnation is explained accordingly: 'Embodied feeling is no longer a medium in which we relate to what we recognize as rightly bearing an aura of the higher; either we do recognize something like this, and we see reason as our unique access to it; or we tend to reject this kind of higher altogether, reducing it through naturalistic explanation.' Put differently, 'The modern development is what we have been calling "excarnation", in particular the exaltation of disengaged reason as the royal road to knowledge, even in human affairs. The proper road to knowledge is by objectification, even in history; [...]. By "objectification", I mean grasping the matter studied as something quite independent of us, where we don't need to understand it all through our involvement with it, or the meaning it has in our lives. The past [or even future, as Marcel seems to posit] is thus another country, and our "objective" understanding of it might be that of anyone, whether they descend from this past or not. We should grasp it in "a view from nowhere"'. (Charles Taylor, *A Secular Age* (Cambridge: Belknap, 2007), 288, 746).

66 Emil M. Cioran, *On the Heights of Despair*, trans. Ilinca Zarifopol-Johnston (Chicago: University of Chicago Press, 1992), 16.

67 Marcel, *Mystery of Being (I)*, 18–38.

68 Terence Sweeney, 'Against ideology: Gabriel Marcel's philosophy of vocation', *Logos* 16, no. 4 (2013): 179–181.

69 Julia Urabayen Pérez, 'El humanismo trágico de Gabriel Marcel: el ser humano en un mundo roto', *Estudios de Filosofía*, no. 41 (2010): 35–59 (37). Translation is mine.

70 Ibid., 37. Translation is mine.

Chapter 1

PAIN, SUFFERING AND THE BROKEN WORLD

People suffer pain. People suffer from broken bones and from broken hearts. People suffer from lesions and from loneliness. People suffer from pain and from the absence of pleasure. And pain is concrete. After all, pains 'can't exist without someone feeling them'.[1] Yet for those experiencing pain, it might also be felt even when there is no physical evidence.[2] And not all pain causes suffering. That is to say, while it is often discussed in relation to pain,[3] suffering does not always as neatly to correspond. Suffering, after all, 'is not merely a matter of pain and other physical symptoms, but in addition has psychological, existential, and social dimensions'.[4] Suffering, accordingly, tends to confound simple clarification and explanation.[5] Moreover, while it might not originate from pain or from illness, 'it [suffering] can make us feel ill and can even cause us to develop various ailments'.[6] So, pain can be a cause of suffering. Yet not always. Suffering can cause further affliction too, heaping burden upon burden.[7]

Nevertheless, people in pain, experienced physically or psychologically or inexplicably, report 'suffering from pain when they feel out of control, when the pain is overwhelming, when the source of the pain is unknown, when the meaning of the pain is dire, or when the pain is apparently without end'.[8] As Eric Cassell has commented further, suffering occurs when persons perceive their pain 'as a threat to their continued existence – not merely to their lives but their integrity as persons'.[9] Such threat can excite experiences of despair. And despair, as Gabriel Marcel proposes, entangles or entraps persons in an unpredictable dialectic that moves between desire and fear; between things not yet possessed and things possessed at risk of being lost.[10]

Suffering, therefore, includes the subjective experience of losing or risking the loss of some perceived good.[11] But those things not yet possessed and those things possessed at risk of being lost, those values in late modern vernacular, are shaped to some degree by 'the character of society [...] [that] determines the way [persons] experience their own physical aches and hurts as concrete pain'.[12] Ivan Illich goes on to clarify, stating that 'The act of suffering always has a historical dimension'.[13]

The historical dimension includes, in part, one's personality. Yet, for those of us shaped by a late modern imagination, the historical dimension also includes those features incumbent to (although not reducible to) the technological age – features that shape human persons and the ways they not only say but also see the world. Technology, after all, 'is entrenched in our history'.[14] Technology demands we attend to it, even if our only relation to it is through refusing or eschewing particular artefacts and applications.[15] Therefore, I want to examine our technological age in which persons continue to grow old and die. Such an examination might help to situate not only pain and suffering experienced by persons in general, but also those persons in later life and confronting irremediable disease, who have also been conformed by late modern *imaginaries* that nurture a secularising 'faith in the efficacy of science [and technology] to alleviate suffering and to cure its ills' – to gain escape from pain and suffering.[16]

To be clear, 'imagination' is what gives shape to our world. Charles Taylor posits that realities exist the way they do *because* of how they are imagined. 'Imaginaries' produce the world in which we live, individually and socially.[17] Accordingly, imagining modernity through a technological gaze and a corresponding rationality has had profound influence on the way we relate to things (and to each other and ourselves as things), including pain, suffering and the like (ageing and dying, for example). The production of our technological age has transformed our experiences of pain and the 'uniquely human performance called *suffering*'.[18] Of course, one must remain aware that technology is not the only transforming power, if you will. Modern sociology has shown time and again the Western project since the Enlightenment has been a project of scientific, technological, legal and political rationalisation committed to 'making life and the world calculable, manageable, and predictable'.[19] Of course, one risks being overly reductive when focusing on technological rationalities. Yet technological imaginaries, corresponding with scientific discoveries, have transformed our expectations that pain and suffering can and therefore ought to be reduced or eliminated. After all, 'the isolation of morphine and acetylsalicylic acid and the arrival of effective surgical anaesthesia in the nineteenth century gave impetus to the supposed "conquest of pain"'.[20] Such management of and the pursuant conquest over pain and suffering has, thus, become 'synonymous with progress', which follows the modern dogma that we 'can in principle master all things by calculation'.[21]

I reflected on that transformation while sitting vigil. Twenty-four hours after haemorrhagic stroke, my mother became unresponsive. Her prognosis was grim and surgical interventions were discussed as unproductive, or futile, given the severity of damage. She was moved from hospital to hospice in a relatively short sequence. Without nutrition or hydration, the focus of the palliative doctors and nursing teams at both institutions focused on expert facilitation of bedside care (repositioning, washing, etc.) and controlling symptoms that might indicate discomfort or pain while she died. At hospice, nursing staff focused on suppressing the gurgling, or death rattle, as she breathed, respirating her final breaths those several days during that final week she laid dying. But in that instance, the clinical focus seemed less to be on my mother and more towards my father and me – they would push anticholinergic medicines[22] to subdue the amount of mucus she was producing in addition to the normal activities of repositioning and mouth care and opioids. While they were attentive to my mother, there was a recurrent concern on us and their perception that such noisy breathing was discomforting or unsettling. Her gurgling was a problem that they could fix. Yet we remained realistic about her state and were not bothered by the gurgling that is a common sign of dying. That such gurgling does not obstruct respiration was known to both my father and me. Yet it seemed that we might have been considered as any of the other 66% of loved ones who find such noise distressing.[23] Overall, however, the disposition among the healthcare teams was towards controlling the environment such that neither my mother nor my father and I would '*suffer* discomfort or distress', as the physicians and nursing professionals would repeat.

And it was in hospice, experiencing grief and unexpected loss, that I began thinking again about Ivan Illich's *Medical Nemesis* and thinking also about a book on technology I had recently finished writing. Regarding the former, I recalled his introduction to 'The Killing of Pain', where he posits that our technological age (what he calls cosmopolitan or medical civilisation) turns everything, including pain, into a kind of problem 'that can be managed or *produced* out of existence'.[24] And I thought the imagery offered was consonant with the way Gabriel Marcel had delimited 'problems' and grieved the broken 'world of the problematical'.[25]

For Marcel, a problem is that which sits as an object of study; something that is set apart or in front of an observer to be surveyed, manipulated and mastered. A problem, like pain, for our late modern imagination, is as any *thing* thrown out in front of us as an obstacle to be resolved. Objectified in that way, pain is as any of the things that we *have* that can either be put to use or disposed of – inert possessions that remain in reserve awaiting consent or contempt. Where one can use pain for a given end, persons find use for it (consider, for example the troubling, instrumental logic of torture). Where one cannot instrumentalise pain to achieve desired aims, technological rationality determines that it ought to be displaced or removed. Pain that corresponds to illness or to injury, for example, in our technological milieu, becomes as any object of knowledge; a thing we have and against which we can learn to exercise control. But without purpose (or as an interference to achieving one's desires), pain becomes an object of disdain, a disvalue.[26] Pain becomes that obstacle or problem which ought to be dispatched. Suffering too?

Suffering is experienced by persons shaped by ways of living and being in the world. It involves, to some significant degree, a judgement that aspects of one's present experience of life is 'intensely negative in nature'.[27] Suffering is often conceived as a disvalue to be minimized.[28] Such judgements reveal from where one might be situated. We might be situated, however, by several (perhaps rival) narratives, histories that delimit how we see and relate with the world. Yet we are all situated by technology too. Suffering like pain, situated by technological imaginaries, is a problem to resolve – it is without meaning save for its standing as a negative stimulus for positive human response.[29] The following helps to illuminate such meaning.

Therefore, I want to think briefly about how we are enveloped not only by artefacts of technology but also by particular technological rationalities that persist and discipline a knowledge of being in the world and, therefore, the meaning of pain and suffering too. As already stated, such focus does not preclude the other imaginaries incumbent to modern processes and paradigms that favour rationalisation and the corresponding efforts 'to make the world controllable'.[30] Yet such focus does raise a particular question, which might be phrased this way: How do technological imaginaries discipline a knowing of (meaning of) and agency towards (response to) both pain and suffering? However, phrasing a question as such is not sufficiently delimited for this digest of sorts. The concepts of pain and of suffering are complex and the experiences of those persons struggling through pain and suffering remain highly particular. Such concepts and experiences deserve and have been subjects of dedicated essays and monographs. Moreover, exploring the panoply of domains where technology pervades and persists in late modern human life would also be an impossibility for one small volume.

Yet provoked by my encounter with Gabriel Marcel, and influenced by thinkers like Ivan Illich and continuing to reflect on my mother and her death, among other influential persons and experiences, the following focuses on the way the technological age has disciplined a perspective on pain and suffering, relative to the medicalized management of life and death. It examines the ways that control, a principal late modern *imaginary*, orients persons' perceptions and responses concerning pain – training us to think of pain 'as a kind of incomprehensible calamity, like a flood, against which we ought to be able to build a dyke'.[31]

The calamity of pain, of course, is incomprehensible because in a world of manipulable *things*, all that ought to be before us is the world of our own making – a world made, suited to our desire. Yet some dykes cannot stem the rising tide of raging waters – an actuality that can excite both fear and suffering. The audacity of suffering, therefore, for those conformed by technological imaginaries highlights the vulnerability to despair, which orients the critical theme of this book. A despair that exposes the inevitable nihilism cultivated, in part, by a technological imaginary[32] – a late modern nihilism that repeats '*Our* pessimism: the world does not have the value we thought it had [...] it seems worth less'.[33]

After all, a world that does not suit our desires, the technological imaginary instructs, is a world that ought not to be.[34] Therefore, the following introduces the technological age as a kind of training, which shapes the way persons come to see the world, including both pain and suffering as problems to resolve. Such training influences the way persons come to know of human being and desire, resulting in a kind of agency disciplined towards control. Such agency, however, leaves persons at risk, vulnerable to the despair that remains coupled to a kind of *hope* the technological, late modern age engenders.

Desiring Control in the Broken World

Leo Tolstoy's *The Death of Ivan Ilyich* offers an account of the final experiences and contemplations of a dying man. A dying man, Ivan Ilyich, is coerced by pain and discomfort, by the depredations that nag and gnaw at him during a protracted end. The imagery of such pain and discomfort is not lost on the reader. But Tolstoy's Ilyich also offers us an account of his pain, which is not only an account of physical frailty and finitude but also an interrogation of the power and limits of medicine and of meaning: 'Is there any meaning in my life that will not be destroyed by the inevitable death awaiting me?'

This is an interesting question prompted by a kind of critical life-reflection as Ilyich realises there is nothing his doctors can do to relieve his pain and that the life he has cultivated is without succour for his final moments. Yet pain, in a technological age, isn't to be that catalyst for such life-reflection. It has become but a disvalue that ought to be minimized. Or, for those who are dying, it is a disvalue from which such persons have a so-argued right from which to be free.[35] Thus, it seems to be of common parlance and disposition that pain is an indignity not fitting of modern subjectivity – not fitting for a world of our having and making. Pain ought to be displaced from the experiences of living and dying. That is to say, pain is meaningless and ought to be removed from our modern human experience.

Put simply, pain is some*thing*, which we do not *want*.

And today, it has been claimed, there are few reasons for a conscious patient to die while experiencing physiological pains she does not want to experience.

Eric Cassell commented nearly two decades ago, it is, as a matter of practice, *easy* 'nowadays to control pain (particularly in hospital and hospice), as well as the efficacy and safety – at least in the short run [...]'.[36] Medicated with a ladder of palliatives from non-steroidal anti-inflammatory drugs to opioids and without pain, patients might be able to live and die unburdened. So, unlike Tolstoy's Ilyich, while his physicians could do nothing to relieve his pain, our physicians work diligently today to snuff out pain and other signs of discomfort – abiding not only a patient's aims but also a modern ideal: control.

Of course, such a death, under the dutiful watch of a palliative care team attending to the slightest upticks in evident pain, or giving competent patients, themselves, control over the mechanised drip of opioids and other palliatives, is a fiction for much of the world. Prevalence of pain for older, dying adults is not insignificant: persons continue to experience pain in the last months, even years, of living,[37] where such experiences can be felt as disruptive (even when under control) and severe[38]; pain can become increasingly exaggerated for terminally ill persons[39]; and problems with chronic pain among many older adults continue un- or insufficiently attenuated.[40] Moreover, the *Lancet* Commission on Palliative Care and Pain Relief has reported unmet palliation for children and adults in many jurisdictions but especially in low- and middle-income countries worldwide.[41] Impoverished persons continue to die in pain, receiving little benefit from advances in the techniques (whether through opioid medications or palliative care) of pain management. Research reveals also troubling racial disparities in not only the recognition of but also the analgesic treatment for pain.[42] Of course, attentive to unmet needs for pain control, the 'ruthless marketing' of OxyContin[43] and other opioid-based products as well as the now-defunct American Pain Society's promotional campaign regarding pain as 'the 5th Vital Sign'[44] has led to the over- and mis-prescription of opioids, contributing to the much-publicised, tragic rise in opioid addiction and related, often deadly[45], crises. (These are realities, I think, that exaggerate 'Modern pessimism [which] is an expression of the uselessness of the *modern* world'.[46]) But such discussions and failures to imagine a just distribution of the abundance of medicines available for pain management are not our present concern. That we don't *want* to experience pain and think that we ought not to experience pain is of concern.

But what of suffering? That question is a bit more challenging to address. To do so, let us retreat to examine pain and the desire for control in our technological age further:

While Hans Jonas might argue technology is ubiquitous in our late modernity,[47] a difficult claim to challenge with smart devices and digital algorithms pervading nearly every aspect of our daily lives, George Grant would argue technology is an ontology.[48] That is to say, technology shapes the way we understand the world and everything in it. Ultimately, Grant's argument of technology is concomitant with Marcel's understanding of the broken world where problems persist and where persons are seduced by 'technological achievements [that] tend to seem more and more the chief, if not the only, mark of man's superiority'.[49]

Technology is not merely a concept or construction. It is not reducible to artefacts of industry or information. It is, rather, a way of seeing, imagining and being in the world. Technology, as such, introduces a kind of pedagogy that disciplines industrial, political and moral life, instrumentalising knowing for the purposes of doing – 'to assure the achievement of some definite concrete purpose'.[50] It disciplines by time and repetition a particular preoccupation with 'having a power over'[51] our problems, while training persons to see all things as material for control.

Let me explain further[52]: Northrop Frye explains why it is, for example, drawing our attention to three modalities of language and their relation to each other, we turn to literature to shape our vision of human civilisation. The first modality regards awareness – the seeing of *things*. Language is used to describe the world before us and set over us. Nouns and adjectives are important here, as they are used to colour and contour what it is that we see. For Frye, at this level of language usage, the world described might have shape and meaning, yet it is not yet a human shape or meaning. The world is viewed from a distance, empirically and objectively (viz. scientifically); perhaps similar to the way in which Marcel speaks of problems, as previously introduced. As a problem, the world puzzle, if you will, stands at our side or in our front readied to be resolved by intellect, ingenuity and industry. Accordingly, it is thought that the objects of awareness or consciousness remain amoral or neutral until ordered by the valuation of the onlooker. At this level of language, the critical reflection about such *things* gives opportunity for the expression of desire: this [adjective] [noun] is not what I want.[53] *That* is a problem that needs to be fixed to suit my desire(s) (or to assuage my fears) – that which I do (or do not) want to see in the world.

The second and third modalities introduce verb forms, which move or orient desires and ideas (our imaginings), respectively. Regarding verbs, actions are essential.[54] The second level introduces us to the means and measures, human activities and automations that will shape the world. This is the level of language where technology, or what Frye calls practical sense, is illuminated: it is needed in order to *accomplish practical aims and achievements*.[55] But the second modality depends on imagination, that is, the third modality. One must have a direction towards which the practical sense can be oriented: 'The world you *want* to live in is a human world, not an objective one: it's not an environment but a home; it's not the world you see but the world you build out of what you see'.[56] It is the third modality, which is literary – introducing and invoking the world we want to have.

We thus begin to say *the world as it does not suit our desires*. The objective world, a constellation of malleable things, is not to our liking. And such valuation is shaped by our imagination. We thus put our practical senses to work, shaping a world to fit our desires; describing it again in its new iteration. Both levels of language, the first and the third for Frye, converge at the technological level, orienting and habituating behaviours that are responsive to both desires and imaginings. The second modality makes of masters, enabled by metaphor and machine, to work *against* the nature we see while seeking to construct a civilisation that satiates our desires and placates our fears. Human beings begin to understand themselves as those capable to recognise and to shape not only nature but also personal experience and social order. Nature, self and society are but structures fit for a rationalist design that persons are capable not only to explain but also to erect.

For our present discussions, Frye's languages might work like this: Pain is concrete. I don't like pain. Pain is not what I want. I can imagine a world without pain. Let us organise knowledge and direct our efforts in order to relieve pain from the human experience.

But how do we come to imagine such a world?

It is the promise and production of power that makes (late) modern technology different from a pre-modern understanding of *technē* and the art or excellence of tool usage. Emmanuel Methene suggests that the possession of power in our present age is what makes modern technology new. But the ontology, the conformation that accompanies the pursuit and performance of such power acquisition, convinces us that we 'can aspire to be free of the tyranny of physical nature'[57] – a physical nature limited by frailty and time that haunts us all. The late modern person is, thus, convinced that humanity either has or ought to have the capacity to shape all things to form, including the experiences and expression of human life. Technology, then, reflects those capacities and the constellation of knowledge arranged for the purpose of accomplishing practical aims and achievements. Such accomplishments and achievements procured to date, however, make it difficult to criticise without being disparaged. That we have means to palliate physical experiences of pain engenders for the late modern person a feedforward trust in technology delimited as such – the commodities of technology procured through the power of an artefact of technology exaggerate further confidence in the power of technology.

Such trust is a trust in the power of technology (the organisation and implementation of our knowledge) to secure our desires. 'Technology' becomes a kind of creed we repeat when encountering the challenges of this life, including the finitude and frailty of a corporeal body that experiences pain – conventionally, as Martin Heidegger suggests, we think of technology as (a) a means to an end and (b) a human-directed activity.[58] Theologically, technology in this way, embodies a heterodox *self*-reflection while a Pelagian anthem, that echo of a modern desire to shape the world to suit ourselves, is rehearsed: by our own desire, rationality and procedure, we will make or appropriate nature, including human nature, accordingly. We can save ourselves and bring relief to the human condition.[59]

Pain as a Problem

The desire to be free from pain while sick or dying, to be free from pain that accompanies losses and loneliness too, is just another desire, an expression of self-determination, which late modern persons trust technological rationalities and the incumbent agencies can (and ought to) resolve. After all, pain is a *problem* to resolve.

Concerning the ought, while moving beyond mere desire, Ivan Illich commented in his *Medical Nemesis*, 'the necessity to bear painful reality, within or without, is interpreted as a failure of the socio-economic system, and pain is treated as an emergent contingency which must be dealt with by extraordinary interventions'.[60] The objective meaning of pain, therefore, has no human meaning, but is positioned as meaningless – pain has no instrumental means, by which humanity can put it to work (except, perhaps, where the illusions of torture as productive persist – thus, at CIA black sites, prison isolation units and other such institutions or insurgencies where brutality is thought useful). Thus, for many of us, we only see pain in its negative form; as an ignoble object to be removed from the body we have and the civilisation being built. Pain becomes the problem which the late modern practice of medicine, with incumbent corporate-scientific, pharmacologic and biotechnological enterprises, can and, therefore, must look to resolve.

And to be sure, when I visit the dentist or require surgery, for example, I am grateful for both the prevention and the relief from pain.

But the point I am making is this: because pain is viewed similarly to every *thing*, as an object, the logic of technological imaginaries persists. Technology *enframes*[61] even the experiences of concrete pain. And by enframing, I am simply repeating, to some degree, George' Grant's claim above; that technology is an ontology, which describes the determinative meaning-making that technology proffers. Technology thus trains us to imagine nature and our experiences of nature as malleable and makeable – even ageing and death, as the following chapters take up. For Marcel, such perspective is indicative of the technocratic character that illustrates the world of the problematical. When the object of our awareness is proven to be an object without use, when it does not fit into the icons and images of desire, it is to be discarded (even if that *thing* is our body[62]). Therefore, the object, including 'objects' of human experience, become enframed by purpose, which is not natural but commodified. It is not mere conscious observation but a disciplining of one's world into a constellation of (actual and potential) problems.

Here we are reminded again of Mesthene's definition that technology is to be delimited as an organisation of knowledge for the purpose of accomplishing practical aims and achievements. Accordingly, the essence of technology in our modern world is not reducible to particular means or artefacts, as one might conventionally understand (technology is not reducible to your iPhone, an industrial machine, or a fleet of autonomous vehicles). Rather, both the Mesthene's definition above and Martin Heidegger's concept of 'enframing' introduce us to an understanding of technology that 'makes modern ingenuity and industry possible by revealing a world where *everything* is observed as a raw material awaiting [organisation and] meaning-making activity – waiting, standing at the ready, to be used for a purpose (or waiting with unremitting anxiety to be discarded as purposeless)'.[63]

Technology, therefore, becomes a practiced posture; persons become conformed to see *things* and prioritise the possibilities of world-making. Through such practiced repetition of technological imaginaries, persons become overcommitted to a kind of homogenous knowing-making pattern that seeks to control all *things*, enframing to form and function for a purpose imposed against objective problems – so we can will to manufacture the world we want to have.

Trusting Technology, Achieving Control over Pain

The modern world is, in part, a technological world – a technocracy.[64] The aims of such a technocracy seem fitting for a modern world committed to controllability. It makes sense then to encounter ways of thinking and doing and being in the world that suit – even when it comes to the human awareness and response to pain. The biomedical or neurophysiological approach to pain management might serve as an example of the ontology encountered.[65] Such an approach identifies the brain as the locus of pain. While the onset of a pain stimulus occurs in the periphery, the nervous potentials ascend to the brain where sensation and perception occur. Physicians thus labour, for example, to identify the objective cause(s) of pain and take advantage of their understanding of the neurotransmitter mechanisms that transmit nervous potentials along the ascending pathways, relieving the brain of sensory and perceptive awareness. The body, in such an approach, is an organism,[66] an organisation of functions that can be identified, assessed and manipulated. When the body, conceived biomedically in this way, presents with disordered functions, that is, pain, the physician labours to re-order the body according to the normative ideal – a pain-free body determined as such by various 'materialistic parameters of measurement'.[67] Pain is therefore treated accordingly.

While many dismiss the biomedical approach as mechanistic, such a way of thinking is not uncommon. In fact, it retains relevance in thinking about pain management. And the clinical categorisation of pain-patients into a medical/physiological classification (rather than psychological, for example) adds further support of the approach.[68] Regardless of classification, the principal aim is to control the experiences of pain. Such control is valued. Such control, it is argued, can be achieved as one comes to possess further knowing. Rather, such control ought to be achieved. And the moral normativity of such an achievement is not only conditioned by an instrumental calculus but also, for example, by rights-based language that presents freedom from pain as a dying persons' *right* (a right which biomedical and nursing professionals are professionally obliged to respond and to secure on the dying person's behalf).[69]

Eric Cassell is critical of biomedical approaches. He argues that a significant issue of contemporary medicine is the way physicians have been trained to focus on discrete diseases rather than on patients; seeing dysfunctions as either physical or psychological, for example, is ultimately a hindrance – especially when attempting to understand pain.[70] For Cassell, pain is not neatly objective, but subjective because it is experienced and expressed by a subject. The person in pain dramatically affects the way the pain is perceived, experienced and expressed.[71] To explain the subjective phenomenon, one could put it this way: while identical in neurophysiological origin and explanation, what one person might experience as a tolerable pain due to a particular chronic illness, another might consider such pain excessive – even to the point of suicidal ideations. (Or, 'it can never be a good argument, in assessing someone's suffering from a certain disease, to say that other people who are in exactly the same physiological condition, do not suffer, or do not suffer severely'[72]). The difference in appreciation, here, as Cassell and others argue, rests in the *awareness* an individual has towards the chronic illness. And for Cassell, such awareness can be changed.

But, as Frye explained above, awareness draws upon both nouns and adjectives and culminates in expressions of desire. It is the imaginative language that invites a perception of meaning about what could be. This is where Cassell's humanistic approach and the biomedical approach converge, both disciplined by a modern, technological imaginary. Control remains preeminent. While the individual person matters, and the particular experiences and expressions of pain ought to delimit both diagnostic and therapeutic plans (rather than a disease condition),[73] each person ought to be given, as a function of their role in the therapeutic relationship, the autonomy or authority over the goals of care.[74] While Cassell's humanistic turn has had great effect upon the thinking about subjectivity (and his work here is vitally important), the end aim remains the same – control. Controlling pain increases one's sense of achievement.[75] The function of exercising control is what makes life meaningful.

But some pains cannot be domesticated. Sometimes pain cannot be subdued by technique. Sometimes the subjective experiences of pain persist unabated.

What then?

Out of Control: Despair Replacing Trust

Unwanted pain in the technological age is made meaningful by its absence (whether objectively, or subjectively). Painlessness, or pain under control, validates a principal value the late modern subject strives towards, the capacity to exert control – and control over things possessed and things desired. The anthropological assumption is that the human being ought to be free to be as she wants to be in the world – the concrete, powerful, self-conscious agent, as I have introduced previously. Such freedom corresponds to ideations about health and success.[76] Thus, the conformed imaginary is that persons should be free from the depredations of corporeality, free from looking at the parts of the world we do not like or want, including pain which, like our frailties and sicknesses, is but an antecedent of death. Pain signifies a deviation from our imaginative ideals of successful ageing. Pain signifies a deviation from healthfulness that is, for biomedicine, defined negatively by absence of dysfunction/disease and positively by totality (health is not merely the absence of disease but also *complete* physical, mental and social well-being).

But not all pains are controllable. Not all can be domesticated, as I exclaimed above. Chronic or unexplained pain, for example, includes a range of adverse consequences for physical and psychosocial function as well as overall well-being. Where those persons evaluate their chronic, or unexplained, pain as an injustice, suffering is enhanced and so is the risk and experience of despair.[77] Such perception of suffering and experience of despair complicates further treatment outcomes – and can lead to ideations of voluntary dying (i.e. suicide). But such perception and risk are incumbent to the way persons are conformed in and by the technological age.

It has been argued that life is meaningful in relation to those values or ideals that one pursues – or as Frye argues, the nature we see and the world we make. We value the exercise of self-determination and competencies of control, not only over nature but also over human nature. We value technological rationalities which organise our knowledge so that we might resolve particular problems and pursue practical aims; so that we might secure the commodities and construct the civilisation of our desires. Yet such meaning-by-values, as such, become susceptible to meaninglessness when such problems prove irresolvable or such aims prove unreachable. Such vulnerability risks feelings of meaninglessness. Such meaninglessness can be realised when the values for which we struggle are not there: one aims but achieves *nothing*.[78] Despair thus emerges.

In medicine, for example, self-determination and the powers of technology to control pain and other experiences of finitude, including the depredations of ageing and dying, are such values for which both physician and patient struggle. Yet in the face of irremediable diagnoses, unrelenting frailties and futile interventions where the modern desire to control is frustrated, meaning is challenged. If one cannot exercise her capacity for self-determination, or the institution of medicine cannot wield its power for controlling the mechanics of living, including the palliation of pain, then the ideals that have previously made life meaningful are dissolved of their value. And despair is the resulting pessimistic apprehension that one's aims have proven illusory: 'that the most powerful desires of life that have the most future have hitherto been slandered', Nietzsche would say, 'so a curse weighs on life'.[79]

To be clear, the late modern vulnerability to despair in our technological age begins with the possibility of realising that which we value, including healthfulness, freedom from pain and control over one's life, but it concludes that we cannot. This conclusion casts persons towards the depths of despair,[80] which is a dialectic of suffering both 'fear and anxiety'.[81] Or as Gabriel Marcel argues, such despair holds persons in an unstable pattern of fear and desire, between things not yet possessed and things possessed at risk of being lost.[82] Sickness, pain, exhaustion, lack of control, depredations and dysfunctions not only exaggerate such fears but also aggravate our desires. Despair antagonises human existence in that way. And it tempts relentlessly until 'One cannot separate the thought of [hopeless struggle] from that of weariness and death'.[83]

The Audacity of Suffering in a Broken World

While Cassell argues experiences of pain do not exclude a kind of hermeneutic, namely a person's interpretive framework (conditioned by a range of factors), suffering and the experiences of suffering, in part, are influenced by cultural categories.[84] Charles Taylor reminds his reader that modern persons desire their lives to be fully satisfactory and want to progress constantly towards a complete sense of fullness – a sense that depends upon the capacities to choose or to control life circumstances.[85] The cultural categories and the constellations of desire and fear are disciplined in our age by technological rationalities and the potentialities to control the experiences and expressions of life – including the experiences and expressions of pain.

Our late modern, technological culture has succeeded in convincing persons that suffering and pain are entirely technological problems to resolve which can be defined exhaustively and treated or prevented by pursuing various means.[86] Yet, as we have considered, when such means prove their futility, persons are left confronted by a threatening meaninglessness of the cultural categories, values, or ideals, that have delimited and defined their pursuits – including the right to be free from pain, for example. And existential suffering persists: 'The experience of existential suffering in modernity therefore expresses a disillusioning confrontation with the facticity of existence that is based on a loss of ability to share the public interpretations of existence and existential demands embodied in modern Western culture'.[87]

A late modern anthropology (coinherent to a technological imaginary) predominates our thinking in the West. It conforms the desires of persons to value self-determination, control and the like. Such an understanding of being in the world trains persons to aim towards a particular expression of autonomy as an ideal. Yet human limitations and functional losses, which are either caused by or produce painful experiences, confound the ideal. Put differently, as Anthony Giddens assesses, self-sufficiency has become a principal doctrine that delimits and defines the human subjectivity in our late modern period; but when conditions of pain or experiences of suffering persist, 'the dilemma of powerlessness [...] has its pathologies [...] and we may speak of a process of *engulfment*. The individual feels dominated by encroaching forces from the outside, which he is unable to resist or transcend'.[88] 'From the outside' might be thought similarly to Frye's introduction of the first level of language and a kind of awareness of phenomena – one sees these encroaching forces, like pain and suffering, as inhuman forces (i.e. not of human desire or form) and expresses disdain.

More than disdain, the person sees the world as it is and expresses that it ought not to be as such. The world ought not to include experiences of unwanted or unrelenting pain. The world ought not to include suffering as a condition of existence. Yet when these valuations of awareness confront the futility of our imaginative functional hoping conditioned by technological rationalities (i.e. I hope that pain can be removed from human experience) and human agency (i.e. I hope that medical scientists and physicians can bring relief), experiences of despair emerge – heaping burden upon burden.

The meaning of pain and suffering in the technological age is conditioned by their absence. The meaning of pain and suffering is coerced by a particular preoccupation with agencies of control and the promises of power that correspond to technological progress. However, when progress is stalled, or the desires of our imagination confront the stubborn actualities of existence, that is, frailty and finitude, despair emerges: 'if I am in pain or virtually unconscious, and have no pleasure, I wish to be helped to die'.[89]

The audacity of pain and suffering, these stubborn actualities of existence, assaults our late modern sense of self-hood and insults our technological imaginary. Being, as conditioned in the technological age as reducible to having an assemblage of functions, is offended. Despair antagonises such a human being, tempting it incessantly. Tempting it towards death, anticipating the very destruction of life itself: 'Man is capable of despair, capable of hugging death, of hugging his *own* death'.[90]

Such despair, as discussed thus far, is rooted in the pessimism nurtured by the modern preoccupation with technology and reduction of all things to (potential) problems. A preoccupation that conditions persons to see suffering, loss and pain as not only visibly unattractive but also meaningless. For persons losing control over life and unable to exercise their knowledge to acquire control over a present or persistent problem, for example, despair provokes and coerces such persons – leaving them alone to anticipate suicide: 'I am only what I am worth (but I am worth nothing)'.[91]

Uncontrolled pain and suffering are meaningless in our technological age. This is why Marcel thinks technology (technocracy) is nihilistic. The inability to control our life problems, even in the absence of conventional pain, excites existential anguish, where fear (and desire) leads to despair. That is to say, as Marcel laments, in our broken world, despair seems to flourish among many, including those persons confronting the pains of irremediable disease and impending death as well as those persons for whom old age and senescence are either actualities of daily life or fears of a future inevitability. The following two chapters consider these particular (but not unrelated) life 'problems': ageing and dying.

Notes

1 Mural Aydede, 'Preface', in *Pain: New Papers on Its Nature and the Methodology of Its Study*, ed. M. Aydede (Cambridge: MIT Press, 2005), ix–xvii (x). Although debate persists about the location of these feelings, whether localised in the mind or felt in the affected regions of the body.

2 Kevin Reuter and Justin Sytsma, 'Unfelt pain', *Synthese* 197 (2020): 1777–1801.

3 Laurel Archer Copp, 'The nature and prevention of suffering', *Journal of Professional Nursing* 6 (1990): 247–249; Deborah Moorehead Thorpe, 'Comprehensive pain care: The relief of pain and suffering', *Dimensions in Oncology Nursing* 4, no. 1 (1990): 27–29.

4 Govert den Hartogh, 'Suffering and dying well: On the proper aim of palliative care', *Medicine, Health Care, and Philosophy* 20 (2017): 413–424 (413).

5 A reason why there is much effort to secure effective measures or tools to analyse suffering empirically, perhaps. See Tyler J. VanderWeele, 'Suffering and response: Directions in empirical research', *Social Science and Medicine* 224 (2019): 58–66.

6 Noella Bueno-Gómez, 'Conceptualizing suffering and pain', *Philosophy, Ethics, and Humanities in Medicine* 12, no. 7 (2017): 1–11 (2).

7 While physical suffering can bring pain, existential suffering, or psychological suffering, can involve fear, anguish or anger. It also is accompanied by the judgement that something, an aspect of one's experiences, is not as it should be – it is experienced negatively; and the weight of the load, which suffering introduces, is not wanted (Beth L. Rodgers and Kathleen V. Cowles, 'A conceptual foundation of human suffering in nursing care and research', *Journal of Advanced Nursing* 25 (1997): 1048–1053). Its relation to the etymology of pain, therefore, seems apropos, given pain has corresponded traditionally to penalty or punishment, which persons must suffer or bear; raising questions about justice that feedback to experiences of suffering (M. J. L. Sullivan, et al., 'The role of perceived injustice in the experience of chronic pain and disability: Scale development and validation', *Journal of Occupational Rehabilitation* 18, no. 3 (2008): 249–261; M. J. L. Sullivan, Whitney Scott, and Zina Trost, 'Perceived injustice: A risk factor for problematic pain outcomes', *Clinical Journal of Pain* 28, no. 6 (2012): 484–488.)

8 Eric J. Cassell, *The Nature of Suffering and the Goals of Medicine* (Oxford: Oxford University Press, 2004), 35.

9 Ibid.

10 Paul O'Callaghan, 'Hope and freedom in Gabriel Marcel and Ernst Bloch', *The Irish Theological Quarterly* 55 (1989): 215–239 (218).

11 John Paul II. *Salvifici Doloris*. Apostolic Letters (Rome, 11 February 1984). Accessed September 2020, http://www.vatican.va/content/john-paul-ii/en/apost_letters/1984/documents/hf_jp-ii_apl_11021984_salvifici-doloris.html.

12 Ivan Illich, *Limits to Medicine. Medical Nemesis: The Expropriation of Health* (London: Marion Boyars, 1976), 178.

13 Ibid., 178.

14 Martin Heidegger, *Parmenides*, trans. André Schuwer and Richard Rojcewicz (Bloomington: Indiana University Press, 1998), 86.

15 Ibid.

16 David Morgan, 'Pain: The unrelieved condition of modernity', *European Journal of Social Theory* 5, no. 3 (2002): 307–322 (313).

17 See Charles Taylor, *Modern Social Imaginaries* (Durham: Duke University Press, 2003).

18 Illich, *Limits to Medicine. Medical Nemesis*, 171.

19 Helmut Rosa, *The Uncontrollability of the World*, trans. James C. Wagner (Cambridge: Polity Press, 2020), 23.

20 Grant Duncan, 'The meanings of "pain" in historical, social, and political context', *The Monist* 100 (2017): 514–531 (519).

21 Morgan, 'Pain', 314.

22 Jason W. Boland and Elaine G. Boland, 'Noisy upper respiratory tract secretions: Pharmacological management', *BMJ Supportive & Palliative Care* 10 (2020): 304–305.

23 Harriëtte J. van Esch, et al., 'Understanding relatives' experience of death rattle', *BMC Psychology* 8, no. 62 (2020): https://doi.org/10.1186/s40359-020-00431-3.

24 Illich, *Limits to Medicine*. *Medical Nemesis* , 171; c.f., Thomas S. Szasz, *Pain and Pleasure* (New York: Basic Books, 1957).

25 Marcel, 'Ontological mystery', 28. A brief commentary on Marcel's world of the problematical, the broken world, and those persons who suffer the objectification of the self can be found here: Hernandez, *Marcel's Ethics of Hope*, 4–27.

26 Of course, unless pain is introduced *for the purpose* of curative or palliative intervention, a familiar medical logic with Hippocratic origin: 'greater pain can erase lesser pain' (Bueno-Gómez, 'Conceptualizing suffering', 3).

27 Rodgers and Cowles, 'Conceptual foundation of human suffering', 1050.

28 Although Arthur Schopenhauer, among others, might consider suffering to be the basic state of life – life is suffering; 'misfortune is the general rule' ('Additional remarks on the doctrine of the suffering of the world', in *Parerga and Paralipomena: Short Philosophical Essays*, vol. 2, trans./eds. Adrian del Caro and Christopher Janaway (Cambridge: Cambridge University Press, 2015), 262–275 (262)). Thus, as he argues, we'd all be better to acknowledge that state and to become accustomed to it.

29 See, for example, Didier Fassin's *Humanitarian Reason: A Moral History of the Present* (Berkeley: University of California Press, 2011) in which he discusses the invention and persistent challenge or impediments of humanitarianism (ix), and articulates a humanitarian rationality that labours 'to correct the situation that gives rise to the misfortune of others' (250). Michael Banner offers a critical evaluation of Fassin's thesis here, 'Regarding suffering: On the discovery of the pain of Christ, the politics of compassion, and the contemporary mediation of the woes of the world', in *The Ethics of Everyday Life: Moral Theology, Social Anthropology, and the Imagination of the Human* (Oxford: Oxford University Press, 2016), 82–106.

30 Rosa, *Uncontrollability of the World*, 28.

31 Marcel, *Man against Mass Society*, 70.

32 Ibid., 195–196.

33 Nietzsche, *Will to Power*, 22.

34 Moyse, *Art of Living*, 39–62.

35 Amelia J. Barbus, 'The dying person's bill of rights', *The American Journal of Nursing* 75, no. 1 (1975): 99.

36 Cassell, *Nature of Suffering*, 261. Challenging managing the experiences of chronic diseases and the persistence of pains, of various kinds, therein remains a continued challenge.

37 Julia M. Addington-Hall and Saffron Karlsen, 'Age is not the crucial factor in determining how the palliative care needs of people who die from cancer differ from those of people who die from other causes', *Journal of Palliative Care* 15, no. 4 (1999): 13–19; Norman A. Desbiens, et al., 'Pain in the oldest-old during hospitalization and up to one year later. HELP Investigators. Hospitalized Elderly Longitudinal Project', *Journal of the American Geriatrics Society* 45, no. 10 (1997): 1167–1172; Alexander K. Smith, et al., 'The epidemiology of pain during the last 2 years of life', *Annals of Internal Medicine* 153, no. 9 (2010): 563–569.

38 A. Meaghen Hagarty, et al., 'Severe pain at the end of life: A population-level observational study', *BMC Palliative Care* 19, no. 60 (2020): https://doi.org/10.1186/s12904-020-00569-2.

39 John N. Morris, et al., 'Last days: A study of the quality of life of terminally ill cancer patients. *Journal of Chronic Diseases* 39, no. 1 (1986): 47–62.

40 Arun Kumar and Nick Allcock, *Pain in Older People: Reflections and Experiences from an Older Person's Perspective* (London: Help the Aged, 2008).

41 Felicia Marie Knaul, et al., 'Alleviating the access abyss in palliative care and pain relief—an imperative of universal health coverage: The Lancet Commission report', *Lancet* 2017 (Published online 12 October), https://doi.org/10.1016/S0140-6736(17)32513-8.

42 Peter Mende-Siedlecki, et al., 'Perceptual contributions to racial bias in pain recognition', *Journal of Experimental Psychology: General* 148, no. 5 (2019): 863–889; Salimah Meghani, Eeeseung Byun, and Rollin M. Gallagher, 'Time to take stock: A meta-analysis and systematic review of analgesic treatment disparities for pain in the United States', *Pain Medicine* 13, no. 2 (2012): 150–174.

43 Patrick Radden Keefe, 'The family that built an empire of pain', *The New Yorker* (23 October 2017): https://www.newyorker.com/magazine/2017/10/30/the-family-that-built-an-empire-of-pain; Art Van Zee, 'The promotion and marketing of oxycontin: Commercial triumph, public health tragedy', *American Journal of Public Health* 99, no. 2 (2009): 221–227.

44 The campaign was based on quality improvement guidelines, which were published a year prior to the campaign launch: See 'Quality improvement guidelines for the treatment of acute pain and cancer pain', American Pain Society Quality of Care Committee, *JAMA* 274, no. 23 (1995): 1874–1880. The APA has since been forced to close due to its complicity in the opioid crisis: Chris McGreal, 'US medical group that pushed doctors to prescribe painkillers forced to close', *The Guardian* (25 May 2019): https://www.theguardian.com/us-news/2019/may/25/american-pain-society-doctors-painkillers.

45 Maia Szalavitz, 'Opioids feel like live. That's why they're deadly in tough times', *The New York Times* (6 December 2021): https://www.nytimes.com/2021/12/06/opinion/us-opioid-crisis.html.

46 Nietzsche, *Will to Power*, 23.

47 Hans Jonas, 'Towards a philosophy of technology', Hastings Center Report (February 1979): 34–43 (34).

48 George Grant, 'Thinking about technology', in *Collected Works of George Grant*, vol. 4 (1970–1988), eds. Arthur Davis and Henry Roper (Toronto: Toronto University Press, 2009), 589–606 (605).

49 Marcel, *Man against Mass Society*, 42.

50 Ibid., 61.

51 Marcel, *Being and Having*, 82.

52 The following comes from my discussion about the way persons are conformed to a technological imagination, here: Moyse, *Art of Living*, 103–114.

53 Northrop Frye, *The Educated Imagination*, CBC Massey Lectures (Toronto: House of Anansi, 2002), 3–5.

54 Ibid., 7.

55 Emmanuel Mesthene, *Technological Change: Its Impact on Man and Society* (New York: New American Library, 1970), 25.

56 Frye, *Educated Imagination*, 5. Emphasis is mine.

57 Emmanuel G. Mesthene, 'Technology and wisdom', in *Technology and Social Change*, ed. Emmanuel G. Mesthene (Indianapolis: Bobbs-Merrill, 1967), 57–62.

58 Martin Heidegger, *The Question Concerning Technology and Other Essays*, trans. William Lovitt (New York: Harper & Row, 1977), 4. We've seen such instrumental and anthropological rationality at work, for better *and* for worse, since early 2020, while nation states and health regions labour to control the rise and spread of the severe acute respiratory syndrome coronavirus 2 (SARS-CoV-2), or COVID-19, through a range of epidemiological modelling, public health policy recommendations, legislated injunctions to curb and contour human behaviours and prophylactic immunization (i.e. vaccinations).

59 Gerald McKenny's *To Relieve the Human Condition: Bioethics, Technology, and the Body* (Albany: State University of New York Press, 1997) remains as essential reading here, examining the influences of a Baconian imagination on human aspirations to bring relief from the burdens of human life (and death). See also Rosa, *Uncontrollability of the World*, 5–29.

60 Illich, *Limits to Medicine. Medical Nemesis*, 173.

61 Heidegger, *Question Concerning Technology*, 20.

62 Marcel, *Being and Having*, 82.

63 Moyse, *Art of Living*, 29. Emphasis is mine.

64 Marcel, *Man against Mass Society*, 193–205.

65 Mariet A. E. Vrancken, 'School of thought on pain', *Social Science and Medicine* 29, no. 3(1989): 434–444.

66 In '[…] medical science the corporeal body is both de-contextualized and de-animated. Medical science does not treat persons as such; it deals with human organisms' (James Aho and Kevin Aho, *Body Matters: A Phenomenology of Sickness, Disease, and Illness* (Lanham: Lexington Books, 2009), 77).

67 Alfred I. Tauber, *Confessions of a Medicine Man: An Essay in Popular Philosophy* (Cambridge: MIT Press, 2002), 9.

68 Bustan Smadar, 'A scientific and philosophical analysis of meanings of pain in studies of pain and suffering', in *Meanings of Pain*, ed. Simon van Rysewyk (Cham: Springer International, 2016), 107–128 (112).

69 See Barbus, 'Dying person's bill of rights,' 99.

70 Cassell, *Nature of Suffering*, 261.

71 See David A. Williams and Beverly E. Thorn, 'An empirical assessment of pain beliefs', *Pain* 36, no. 3 (1989): 351–358.

72 Hartogh, 'Suffering and dying well', 415.

73 Cassell, *Nature of Suffering*, 282.

74 Ibid., 283.

75 Ibid., 281. The idea of 'control' is important for Cassell, and is repeated often.

76 For discussions about health and success, see the second and third chapters, respectively.

77 Sullivan, et al., 'Role of perceived injustice in pain and disability', 249–261, 484–488.

78 Nietzsche, *Will to Power*, 12.

79 Ibid., 22.

80 Friedrich Nietzsche, *Thus Spoke Zarathustra*, trans. Adrian Del Caro (Cambridge: Cambridge University Press, 2006), 228.

81 Cioran. *Heights of Despair*, 19.

82 O'Callaghan, 'Hope and freedom', 218.

83 Cioran, *Heights of Despair*, 16.

84 Iain Wilkinson, *Suffering: A Sociological Introduction* (Cambridge: Polity Press, 2005).

85 Charles Taylor, *A Secular Age* (Cambridge, MA: The Belknap Press of Harvard University Press, 2007), 20.

86 David Morris, *The Culture of Pain* (Berkeley: University of California Press, 1993), 2.

87 Anders Dræby Sørensen, 'The paradox of modern suffering', *Tidsskrift for Forskning i Sygdom og Samfund* [*Journal of Research in Disease and Society*] 7, no. 13 (2010): 131–159 (139).

88 Anthony Giddens, *Modernity and Self-Identity: Self and Society in the Late Modern Age* (Cambridge: Polity Press, 1991), 193.

89 Anthony M. Warnes, 'Being old, old people, and the burdens of burden', *Ageing and Society* 13 (1993): 306.

90 Marcel, *Being and Having*, 104; c.f., Gabriel Marcel, *Homo Viator: Introduction to a Metaphysic of Hope*, trans. Emma Craufurd and Paul Seaton (South Bend: St Augustine's Press, 2010), 36–38.

91 Marcel, *Being and Having*, 104.

Chapter 2

AGEING AS 'ONE MORE OPPORTUNITY TO FAIL'

In *A Short History of Decay* Emil Cioran writes of the 'Decrepit Man': 'The time is past when he thought of himself in terms of a dawn; behold him resting on an anemic matter, open to his true duty, the duty of studying his loss and rushing into it [...] behold him on the threshold of a new epoch'.[1] While those persons whose ageing bodies have obliged such learning and haste, the new epoch can bring with it a vulnerability to despair. For Cioran, the *anaemic matter* of an ageing body, 'Having reached the intimacy of [its] autumn, [...] wavers between Appearance and Nothingness'.[2] However, the body in later life also speaks quite actively (and at times quite loudly), revealing in the sounds of creaking and cracking, the actualities of frailty and finitude. It therefore calls out for attention – claiming not only oneself but also others to heed its summons. In this way, the body bares – that is, it *reveals* – the burdens of ageing, which persons (and others) must learn to bear, in the sense of 'carry'. But we, ageing persons, as our bodies, can also labour diligently, even dutifully, to conceal such burdens too – and we often do, not wanting to be(come) a burden on others.

You might be familiar with that decision to conceal burdens. I know that I am, certainly: I was raised on the Saskatchewan prairies. For the uninitiated, it is a place where you learn to work hard in harsh conditions, rarely, if ever, pausing when problems arise and when your body aches or breaks down. After all, the calf must be birthed, even in the middle of the slush of cold mud and freezing rain. Harvest must come in before the freeze, you know – keep working through the day and the night. The worn-out tractor must be repaired to turn over the soil for a late start seeding, ignoring the bloodying of knuckles and cuts upon one's arm as one's limb is contorted to the shape of the engine and the orientation of adjacent rusting metal, because the cost of new machinery is too great and the growing season too short. Back hurting and hands numb, the several feet of snow must be shovelled or ploughed from the drive to liberate your car in time to travel the icy winter roads for work or school – it was an extreme rarity growing up for anything to be postponed because of inclement winter weather. In these conditions, among others, you learn to take pride in your independence to do all of this without voicing complaint and unnecessarily burdening others in your efforts.

Sure, in prairie communities, neighbours will lend a hand in haste and without pomp. The community does gather to bolster one another in Saskatchewan. Yet the celebratory discussions at the concluding hallmarks that fill the calendar rarely include recognition of the inter-dependence that serves as a stark juxtaposition to the predominating celebration of independence.

I've certainly been influenced by these same habits of independence (inheriting a rather stubborn disposition too). Such formation habituated a perspective that one must be fiercely independent – showing capabilities at every turn at the cost of hiding burdens. I am confronted by such a perspective each time I look at the fifth finger of my right hand. I am forced by its kinks and crooks to remember that familiar logic of independence and burden which is often habituated by corresponding practices of alienation (I can do this myself) and denial (I do not want to be a burden), respectively. These are habits not unfamiliar to those one might see practiced by persons in my family, in my hometown and in my province. Such practices are not unfamiliar to the prairies and in so many locations in the Western world.

But you might ask, why that crooked finger?

When I returned home for lunch, after breaking my finger while playing basketball one morning during fifth grade physical education, I revealed to my mother a gnarled phalanx bent in a way that a finger ought not to bend. I grimaced with pride and exclaimed, 'Mom, I didn't tell anyone I broke my finger!' She gathered my hand cautiously, inspected carefully, moved the finger around gently. She enquired about pain. I lied. She praised my grit but expressed that a trip to hospital might be a good idea – she was a nurse, after all, and providing care to others who have been injured was of normal routine. I expressed otherwise and wrapped my finger to its adjacent partner with hockey tape and finished lunch.

Mom then gathered me for a trip to hospital for further evaluation anyway (remember, I've inherited a particular disposition). The doctor observed my finger in a matter-of-fact sort of way, set a joint (that hurt!) and an x-ray was ordered. She pointed out a small fracture, was satisfied with alignment and flatly said I'd be fine. Then, she wrapped my fingers together *with tape* – I gave Mom a look of smug self-sufficiency; my expression of independence was vindicated.

I learned early on while growing up that independence was valued and that it was to be secured without burdening others. Perhaps you did too. At least, many persons do model a similar disposition – never wanting to be a burden and labouring diligently to exercise independence. It is of this value that I want to focus our attention at present. I want us to focus too upon the inverse of the message regarding independence as a principal function to desire, which is this: to be(come) a burden on others is assumed as a disvalue. Dependence is as a dysfunction to fear.

But what constitutes a burden?

For those of us with broken fingers and bodily depredations incurred by corporeal frailties that become increasingly familiar in later life, burdens are bodily phenomena that might make heavy the work of living. Such phenomena might include a painful back, like the father of a high school friend – a excruciatingly painful back, both before and after surgery, that made walking, standing, any posture at all, difficult (and he was not yet 'old' in his years). It might include painful peripheral mononeuropathies, like that of a later-life friend of my parents who visited our house regularly when I was young but struggled to move about proficiently, aided by his walking stick and later his walking frame. It might include painful joints of the hand that make the opening of jars a feat of pain and struggle, as my grandmother experienced each time that she attempted to open the jars that contained her preserves, jams and jellies. Of course, one could conjure any number of examples – these are the pains of older persons I observed while growing up; agonies that each discussed with me, though often with lamentation and grief for experiences of an unencumbered past.

However, not all burdens are borne from flesh and finitude. Some burdens are constructed and laid upon the shoulders of ageing persons further conditioned by preoccupations with independence. I'll say more of such fabricated burdens below. Yet, to be sure, both burdens must be given attention. Both burdens must be confessed and understood considering our present history; a history shaped, in part, by our perceptions of the broken world.

The following will to do just that, setting out frailties in later life, viz. ageing, as a 'problem' of life, which risks despair. Stepwise, I discuss first a late modern anthropology, or understanding of human agency or subjectivity, that predominates in our thinking and acting in the broken world; a kind of disembodied ideal of functional independence overshadowed by the actualities of frailty and finitude. By 'overshadowed', I mean to suggest that such actualities like bodily frailties and the depredations that can occur in later life serve to challenge such a functional ideal, revealing its limit or fiction. Subsequently, the following discusses the burdened self-image that can be cultivated by the experiences and expressions of the ageing person who has become limited by the actualities of corporeality and impacted by socially constructed burdens, familiar to our late modernity. These such limitations and burdens are often potent and coercive, constraining the way persons see themselves and others in the world. The chapter will conclude while focusing on the inclusion of independence as a policy measure that aims towards successful ageing but sustains a kind of 'hope' for a particular agency (or way of vital and social functioning in the world) that renders persons vulnerable to despair – exaggerated by experiences of failure and loss. Such experiences risk a despair that goads persons to evaluate life as it is or as it might become in the future as a life that ought not to be; a life of encumbered agency, of diminished functions, as a life without meaning. Such despair impedes human flourishing and cultivates hopelessness. Accordingly, this chapter will continue the work of discriminating, or diagnosing, the mechanics of despair incumbent to a late modernity that prioritizes particular ideal features, or functions, of the human condition.

The Long Shadow of the Fourth Age

A characteristic of a modern anthropology is often found among policy recommendations for what persons refer to as 'successful' or 'health ageing': it revolves around ideations of independence. Such an anthropological ideal prioritizes functional independence through which persons learn to emphasize self-sufficiency as a vital and social function one ought to have – one should possess the freedom from dependence.

Repeating independence as an essential function, persons are taught that it is right and good to exercise that particular achievement, through which one can come to possess (even master) the freedom to act in the world without constraint or coercion (i.e. autonomy). Of course, autonomy and independence can be analytically differentiated, as one might read in self-determination theory. Where distinctions are held, independence regards the 'circumstances of not relying on others for support, help, or supplies'[3] while autonomy reflects an individual's freedom from 'constraints placed on her behavior as a result of exploitative, unequal, or oppressive conditions'.[4] The opposite of the former is dependence and the latter is heteronomy. These opposites disclose a locus of relation between independence and autonomy. In both antonyms, particular persons relate to others, whether persons or institutions or otherwise, as those or as that which might constrain one's freedoms and determine one's behaviour or access to opportunities. Thus, whether dependence or heteronomy, or perhaps both, the functional capacity to exercise self-determinative control over the experiences and expressions of one's life remains at risk. And such control is considered essential, or basic, by those for whom independence and autonomy are functional priorities to secure.

Independence, autonomy and control might be considered further under the notion of agency, which some might regard as the power or capacity to act.[5] Such an understanding, while contested,[6] remains a common understanding and concurrent with the way the World Health Organization, for example, delimits its Active Ageing policies and programming. Diego Romaioli and Alberta Contarello explain the WHO position thusly:

> The concept of 'active ageing' refers to an ongoing involvement of older people in activities and plays a key role in a global strategy for the management of ageing populations. The notion of activity is understood as an active/passive distinction which emphasises the enhancement or diminishment of *measurable powers of activity*. Active ageing is part of a policy vision that will enable the expanding older population to remain healthy (thus reducing the burden on health and social care systems) and to stay employed longer (thus reducing pension costs).[7]

Both independence and autonomy feed into the understanding many might have regarding agency as the power of particular functions to initiate action while the desires to maintain such capacity are cultivated by the repetition of such values in policies or programmes and the tenets of a modern anthropology.

That the terms remain highly subjective, contextual and definitionally in flux among older persons, however, adds further fodder to the challenges at delimiting clear meaning.[8] Although we can (and will here) accept colloquial interpretations of autonomy and independence, which can and often do conflate or show significant overlap between these terms. Persons in the late modern age do learn that opportunity, choice and control over the circumstances of one's life are essential (even 'innate, instinctual, and unquestionable'[9]) characteristics of agency that one ought to have and that which inhibits such freedoms is a problem to be overcome or to be liberated from. For those persons confronting inhibitions of human finitude, for example, control over the 'landscape of disease',[10] including what some regard as the pathology of ageing, is thought possible and that persons in later life will be enabled to maintain a freedom from a constellation of phenomena like frailty, pain and suffering. Independence is considered as essential to exert or to take advantage of such control and to exercise autonomy.

Put differently, a familiar modern anthropology trains persons to desire for autonomy and to delimit independence as the corresponding ideal, which persons ought to possess. These aims have also shaped policy responses to the challenges of ageing, for example. Such policies foreground independence and individual industry (to pursue available options and to control one's experiences), accordingly. Independence and autonomy have thus risen together as anthropological orthodoxy in late modernity.

'Independence' is, thus, read often in policy statements concerning successful or healthy ageing. Self-sufficiency/self-reliance and control, among other characteristics of agency or synonyms of autonomy, are corollary functions needed to achieve the good life for independent persons conditioned by our late modern imaginaries. (One need only to look at research which reveals the way older persons, including those experiencing frailties, value independence,[11] and resist care from others for various reasons that correspond to valuations of independence,[12] and a persistent patriarchy that divides some from others, the weak from the strong.[13] Policy thus reiterates such aims and hierarchies of being when calling forth 'independence' to guide actionable programming and practices – programming and practices by which persons are further conditioned, in a kind of positive feedback loop, to choose and to consume and to fulfil one's self, as though an outcome of particular functional achievements.

The 'third age' typology or classification of later life seems to emphasize the opportunities available to and the agential successes of those persons that prove capable to secure or to maintain these aims. Such life is defined, so it is argued, by personal fulfilment through the administration of choice over and the freedom to pursue the opportunities made available to persons. 'Independence' in policy statements concerning successful or healthy ageing serve as a synonym of such fulfilment that can be secured through the commodities proffered by a technologically determined and consumer market-driven health-industrial-complex that advertises the promises of self-sufficiency and control as the means towards successful, healthy ageing and rejuvenation.[14] These reiterate the aims that narrate the 'good life' for persons whose lives have been shaped by a modern imaginary where independence and control are correlating concepts or coinhering ideals.

Yet, when these same persons experience threats to or the loss of these characteristics (aims or values), whether expressed as independence, control, self-sufficiency, or the like, experiences of despair emerge. When others consider the threat to or the loss of these characteristics the same diagnostic applies and despair is made further evident. Thus, an existential weight is placed upon persons, whether by their own self-image or by others, as the aims that render meaning for persons prove aimless or illusory.

This existential weight, of course, introduces us to the aetiology of despair. Let me explain: the failure to secure the aims of our desires prove such aims are aimless and the world which persons thought meaningful in relation to such aims proves meaningless – promoting despair. This is akin to the despair Gabriel Marcel has introduced us to previously – despair that emerges from the failure to have that which we desired or feared we might lose. Put differently, Marcel thinks of such despair as emerging from a kind of 'enchantment', served by a 'dismal repetition' that is both present and anticipated as a determinative fate.[15] The repetition might be heard as such: 'I have never been disappointed so many times there is every reason to expect that I shall be again today. [...] I shall never again be anything but the wounded, mutilated creature I am today'.[16] Or, in the words of an 82-year-old male who previously attempted suicide, giving reason for self-harm, the 'dismal repetition' might be heard as such: 'I am not self-sufficient now because I can't walk properly. [...] Wee wee and poo poo, the nurses have to attend to me [...]. Because of stroke, wasn't able to move. Can't even remove my clothing. [...] I am here waiting for death'.[17]

Tempted to such despair, persons are hedged in by anguish.[18] Accordingly, for persons in later life who are (desiring but fear) losing capabilities that correspond to independence, control and self-sufficiency, functional characteristics of the ideal agent, despair can emerge. As it does emerge, it foists an existential weight, an anxiety, upon persons that is experienced as they confront what Peter Laslett calls the 'fourth age'.[19]

While some offer a definitive age when persons enter this stage of life, that is, beginning at around 85 years of age,[20] Laslett argues this stratum of a life-stage is delimited, rather, by the disvalues of a modern imagination, including those *problems* like dependency, decrepitude and death.[21] Such conditions of living rather than a chronology of years-lived delineate the journey towards and into fourth age experiences. Whether a distant fear or as a proximate stressor, the aims that render meaning for a modern imaginary are either threatened or lost in this life-stage, regardless of chronological age. Put differently, the inability to control our life circumstances and to secure self-[functions] (such as self-*reliance*, self-*sufficiency*, and self-*determination*) of agency excites both fear and anguish, burdening one's being while leading to despair. 'Suffering', as the experience of despair, parallel to both Nietzsche and Marcel above, is 'the state in which people are subject[ed] [...] to loss or defects that prevent them from achieving their specific opportunities'[22] – prevented from achieving, for example, the aims or ideals or desired *things* of the third age.

One could highlight several examples where such despair might emerge in our late modern milieu. But Jean Améry's reflections on ageing outline with bleak prose the cost that advanced age brings to the human body, mind and spirit. He suggests the frail elderly come to rest and are forced by the depredations of ageing to make do without (principally, to make do without the capacities to master their world and to shape it to their desires).[23] Similarly, scholars in palliative and health care research have observed that persons confronting unrelenting prognoses and irremediable diagnoses are also forced, by the devastations of disease and dysfunction, to make do without – a focus of the third chapter. Finally, economists Anne Case and Angus Deaton have observed that a subsection of the US population have been forced to make do without as diminishing employment and economic opportunities become fodder for anguish.[24] While experiences of vocational purpose are lost, life becomes burdensome and meaningfulness is obscured, if not experienced as altogether lost. Whether frail elderly, dying or economically distressed, persons in such states of crisis discover themselves to be in a world they no longer understand, experiencing their lives as without the capacities to engage with it – a kind of fourth age experience. They find themselves in situations beyond their control; that control they've laboured to strengthen, to exercise and to secure by commodity and consent. Beyond control, they are turned towards despair. Such despair, as these authors above seem to suggest, generates behaviours that anticipate suicide or other, often tragic, outcomes that impede or greatly curtail or even completely inhibit human flourishing.

And here is where the aims of industry, policy, healthcare practitioners and all of us who are growing older can likely agree: to flourish as a human being is good. So, many of these advances to extend the healthful experiences of later life persons are good too.

Yet the fourth age casts a long shadow over the third age. ('Hence when participants speak of the value of independence and its central relevance to active ageing, they tend to do so against the backdrop of the subjective spectre of dependency – of being an unwanted "burden" on others',[25] contributing to stigmas and stereotypes that serve as fodder for despairing ideations and the cultivation of burdens that are not only borne of ageing bodies but also of social imaginaries (of freedom, control and the like) that can, ironically, coerce and constrain experiences of later life).

I'm not convinced, however, that the promises and powers of our late modern imagination to extend third age experiences into later life do anything to curtail a story about 'being independent', about agency or subjectivity, that leaves us vulnerable to despair. That is to say, while Karen Blixen (using her *nom de plum* Isak Dineson) was attributed to have said 'I think all sorrows can be borne if you put them into a story and tell a story about them', I am not convinced that our late modern story does well to offer us such strength. Instead, I am concerned that a story of late modern agency leaves persons coerced by delusions of independence (of absolute subjectivity). It is a story which leaves persons vulnerable to despair. It is a story that marginalizes experiences of corporeal burdens and the fear-inducing perceptions of being or becoming a burden to others by its predictable re-assertion of late modern values and concomitant policy aims. Yet such a story of late modern agency, and the policy aims it cultivates, remains overshadowed by the looming darkness of the fourth age.

Topologizing Burdens that Constrain Later Life

For many, even while age-specific disability rates seem to be falling among older persons,[26] ageing is expected to include or does involve experiences of diminished everyday competence.[27] As geriatrician Louise Aronson acknowledges, the changes that one encounters as one grows older occur across a long range of time and at a variety of rates, particular to each individual person. Yet, universally, the 'parts of this transformation – the losses – initially require adaptation, then limitation, and sometimes, finally, renunciation'.[28] Such existential changes increase with age.[29] It seems clear, or make sense, the physical encumbrances not excluding psycho-emotional distresses and cognitive decline as well the age-related loss such declines and limitations determine also can be debilitating ontologically. Growing old is a difficult phenomenon to reconcile for persons. In fact, as Els van Wijngaarden, Carlo Leget and Anne Goossensen observe, the vulnerability to despair at the burden of ageing, even in the absence of severe disease, resources a readiness to terminate the life of which persons have grown tired.[30] Iris Hartog and her colleagues, including van Wijngaarden, have added to these findings, observing that while older adults who have grown tired of living might also present with a persistent death wish, not all persons wish, actively, to end their life.[31] But the spectre of meaning in one's life, whether or not life might be(come) meaningless, remains an active question that highlights the shadow of the fourth-age and contributes, with significance, to ideations of suicide (or the prevalence of a death wish).

Nevertheless, studies examined in 'Experiences and motivations underlying wishes to die in older people who are tired of living' point out that age-related losses include the suffering corresponding to 'physical decline and ongoing deterioration of walking, vision, hearing, speaking and sensory abilities, cognitive decline, incontinence and impotence. [...] [deepen] feelings of powerlessness, growing dependency on others, and loss of privacy and control'.[32] Loss of control is thus experienced by older persons as a loss while they rush into it, to draw us back to Cioran's imagery which inaugurated this chapter. Loss of connectedness correlates: 'the sense of being no longer valued, needed or significant provokes feelings of worthlessness, invisibility to others, and detachment from community'.[33]

In another essay, van Wijngaarden, Leget and Goossensen suggest the burden of ageing excites 'significant feelings of disconnectedness, reflected in feelings of loneliness, not mattering, fear of dependence, self-estrangement, and alienation'.[34] Such feelings accompany the self-perception of burden, which delimits the experiences of ourselves *as* old – experiences which, for each one entering later life, are personally or subjectively unfamiliar and unchartered.

These experiences, however, are not simply an existential self-perception of being and becoming older. Such experiences also include the gaze from others, who might be perceived as voyeurs of our decline – contributing to experiences of shame and anxiety (or dread).[35] As such persons can come to regard themselves as once, but no longer, viewed as an individual imbued with the reason and will to possess the world, to control one's life; once, but no longer, viewed by self and others as capable to guarantee self-actualization, achieving what was thought essential and meaningful. One's health, as delimited by an aged and ever-ageing body, often limits such agency while persons are situated further by frailty and finitude; or worse, excluded in ways from which they cannot struggle to reject or to revoke. Such persons, it seems, respond in foreseeable ways. Such persons, disciplined to think about the world (and themselves in it) according to a modern imaginary, come to realize 'the world does not have the value that [they] once thought it had'.[36] Thus, as Nietzsche concludes, it seems to be a world without value – 'worthless'.[37] Or to draw upon the observations of van Wijngaarden and her colleagues, such persons come to a point of pessimism, experiencing desperation and assessing that '*life-as-it-is* [the old life] should stop as soon as possible because of the unbearable burden it embodies'.[38]

But an important question yet remains: what does *burden* mean?

Burden is meant to connote a weight that is carried. It is a familiar connotation. Perhaps it is even fitting, when considering the experiences of bodily life as we grow older: with the depredations of ageing, the burden of one's body can, after all, be experienced as a heavy weight one must overcome to sit up in bed, to stand from sitting and to ambulate from place to place. But defining burden this way, as a weight to carry, continues with figurative allusions, like a distress that is emotionally difficult to carry, or a source of great worry. Our fears and desires can heighten this distress, making relevant the various synonyms of burden, such as 'affliction, cross, [or] trial' (OED). Such nouns are intended to denote something onerous or troublesome, as 'something wearisome or grievous'.[39]

The physical and psychological wearisomeness experienced by persons in later life is a recurrent theme. That is to say, the bodily trials of ageing are described as a burden, reflexively.[40] But the reflexive dirge of the person grieving their losses of competence, self-sufficiency and independence includes a transitive counterpart, expressed, commonly, as 'I don't want to burden others'. This type of burden has two characteristics, which follow the grammatical characteristics of transitive verbs. First, it assumes burden as an action. Second, it has, as its object, someone who will receive the action. In this case, persons who perceive this transitive counterpart to reflexive burden are concerned they will encumber (action) others (object) – they will burden family members, friends, caregivers or others. Put differently, this is where a person's self-perceived burden includes a correlating perspective (or fear) that one is at risk of being a burden for others. People not only experience the burdens of finitude, but also wrestle with the ideations that foreground self-perceptions of being as a burden for others to bear. 'Being "burdensome" would, logically, mean *imposing* or *depending* on others whose assistance or willingness to help cannot be assumed or counted on'.[41] Apprehension and dread, for example, can accompany the prospective experiences of becoming a burden.[42] Fear 'of a long and debilitating fate', where 'I am going to be a burden to anybody', too.[43]

Self-perceived burden, including the reflexive and transitive expressions of burden, resource 'a general sense of suffering' and risks 'clinical depression, a diminished will to live, and a [perceived] loss of dignity'.[44] This perceived burdensomeness can result in 'shame, low self-esteem, and self-hatred'.[45] It is a relevant factor in death-hastening ideations and acts among aging persons, including withdrawing and refusing medical treatment through to suicide and medically mediated death.

But another response is also common: concealing burden. The attempt to 'minimize their own needs', which includes behaviours like 'concealing their feelings or symptoms, not bothering others, withdrawing so as not to cause upset, and to try and do as much as they could for themselves even when this caused discomfort' serves as a vestige of the unencumbered subject. Consider the words of participant ID13, transcribed by Christine McPherson and her colleagues: 'I can hide it. I can mask it. [...] I had learned you could mask a little bit, or you can pretend a little bit, [...] being a great pretender, not in an intentional, misleading way, but protective'.[46] It is not uncommon for frail ageing or sickly persons to conceal the perturbations that make daily life difficult, to protect themselves from feeling like a burden and to protect others from experiencing care-giver burden.

In fact, as McPherson and her colleagues observed, 'Almost all participants had difficulty asking for and accepting help from others, and were reluctant to do so even when needs emerged'.[47] Many see it as a failure when they are unable to perform the social roles that have defined them to date. As ID13 would suggest, transitioning from being an independent and caregiving mother, to a person whose children must give care: 'It's a very difficult transition'.[48] To be(come) a burden on others is assumed as a disvalue. To become a burden, the impact one might have on others, whether relatives, health care professionals, or care volunteers, is in fact feared.[49]

Such fear might be rightly placed: it certainly reflects the difficulty of admitting burden's further usage, which is likely familiar given the *burden narrative* of old age. It is a narrative not about the subjective experiences of growing old, of the hardship experienced when becoming dependent on others against one's will, but the weighted impact of ageing that others claim for themselves or for society.

As Andrea Charise's 'Let the reader think of the burden: old age and the crisis of capacity' argues, catastrophic metaphors are part of a familiar, but unfortunate and coercive, discourse that positions persons of older ages as complicit others:

> The ominous rhetoric of rising, swamping, tides, and disease— amplified by the authoritative tones of medical and health policy expertise—conceives of population ageing as an imminent catastrophe. Conceived *en masse*, the aged are naturalized as a liquid cataclysm whose volume exceeds the nation's ability to contain, or even guard against, an abstracted human burden.[50]

The burden narrative, catastrophically retold, functions by producing 'the elderly population' as a peculiar and delimited political and consumer reference class that threatens both social and economic covenants. Such narratives function as *accusative burdens*, which add further fodder to the burden self-image – an image, as we learned above, that doesn't need any further assistance in demoralizing and debilitating human lives.

The accusations introduce burden as a charge laid '*upon* (a person)', a sense of *burden* included in the OED. It functions when older adults are indicted as the object rather than recognized as the subject of burden. 'What happens is that the agents carrying the burdens are misidentified: the more graphic the portrayal of the wearisomeness of old age, poverty or sickness, the greater the sense of grievous load upon others'.[51] Once again, 'they' are thus catastrophized as a collective social problem with metaphors describing the ageing population as a tsunami or a rising tide, which 'threatens to swamp our health-care system, economy, and quality of life'.[52] Accusative burdens, such as these, reflect those *burdens* often applied to older adults in two ways: first, the financial load incurred by income supports as well as health and social care costs; second, burden is applied to both care-giving efforts and stresses. When applied to a population, that is, the Fourth age, or to a dependent, that is, an ageing parent, 'whatever the intention, *burden* is often demeaning, carrying the implication that the person, and more often the group is a nuisance, wearisome or costly to support'.[53]

Burden in such circumstances is used to connote a sense that such irritants are too much, that ageing might trigger socio-economic and/or intergenerational crises, while goading public reactions that call for such liabilities to be reduced or eliminated.[54] Put differently, the ageing population that threatens such potential catastrophe, so it is argued, demands remediating attention. The accusative assumption is that the burden of societal ageing should be a source of global moral concern and generative of 'remorse rather than pride'.[55] Thus, as the burden narrative gains further prominence, lives of decline and frailty are narrated as *problems* to resolve, or are considered as worthless, while youth and agility are praised. The latter should be considered normative, while the former put to an end, as the controversial *Ending Aging* contends.[56]

And so, people already subjected to the weight of reflexive and transitive burden are further weighed down by a demeaning accusative burden, which only risks exaggerating and perniciously validating one's burdened self-image. The ageing and aged population, this objective reference class, is increasingly risking economic as well as intergenerational and caregiver distress and is marked by others as a burden. That is the accusative burden.

Yet what unites such burdens? What is common among them?

At the very least, a common concern regards the weight that diminishing independence bears on the well-being of those who are growing old. In studying the experiences of burden among older persons, it becomes clear that individual agency, which includes expressions of independence, self-sufficiency and the like, is considered deeply integral to one's identity. However, as a deeply held desire and a necessary condition of late modern human being, the weight corresponding to a particular preoccupation with individualistic and unconditional notion of independence (and corresponding instrumental attitudes in economics) seems to oppose human flourishing.

Independence as Ideal and Affliction

The experience of ageing concerns several things; for Jean Améry, as we enter what some might refer as the fourth age and *become* old, we lose access to space and the world. That is, with a rather pessimistic realism, Améry suggests that the world becomes inhospitable or inadmissible – like mountains we can no longer climb.[57] Put differently, the frail older person, as Améry observes, becomes 'a stratified mass of time'[58] who is increasingly aware of her physicality – but with increasing limitations, it is a physicality that becomes progressively inert. And for some, like Ezekiel Emanuel, introduced previously, the inertia of older age offers him warrant to wish for his death before ageing becomes insufferable. You might recall from the introduction; he wants to die at 75. He anticipates his death at (or soon thereafter) that chronometric age because, by that time of senescence, 'creativity, originality, and productivity are pretty much gone for the vast, vast majority of us'.[59] The losses one experiences or fears, as in Emanuel's case, become fodder for ideations that death might be one's only hope.

While the ageing person experiences increasing losses, they are also met by 'society and everyone's demand for social *self*-preservation'.[60] The ideals of independence, however, confront the realizations that ageing bodies, especially those encumbered by illnesses and frailties, are not self-sufficient, self-determining and strong. Rather, ageing persons can experience, with older age, their bodies as deficient, dependent and delicate: at 72 and having attempted suicide, Mr Z. depicted those who one might consider as old, saying 'Somebody who has false teeth. Somebody who is bald. Somebody who has a walking stick. Somebody who is not terribly astute and on the ball. Somebody who moans and groans and complains. All those sorts of things'.[61] Rather, such persons can discover the body as it is increasingly burdened 'more frequently every day' by age-related depredations.[62] Chris Gilleard and Paul Higgs refer to this experience as 'age's 'corporealisation' – the emergence of bodily signs of ageing'.[63] As the body becomes increasingly ever-present to such persons in new ways, like the discomforting pressures of arthritic joints, or the distressing fatigue of muscles working to climb up a flight of stairs, or the disorienting figments floating in one's field of vision – many such experiences are remediable; yet others remain persistent and irremediable 'existential limitations'.[64] that 'cut us off from the world'.[65]

Such a depiction of older age, while quite possibly overly negative to some, might find analogous descriptions in ageing studies literature. For example, 'the body drop' experienced by ageing persons, as Kevin McKee and Marynn Gott have discussed, highlights the perceived failings of the ideal agent that compound experiences of burdensomeness.[66] 'Events such as a fall, an episode of incontinence, or of erectile dysfunction are examples of such "body drops". [...] the humiliation felt by older people who see such episodes as symbolic of their own, age-associated "failings" *to maintain themselves*', in the world resource the perceived burdensomeness of ageing.[67]

Further fears concerning the potential loss of one's mind, a pre-eminent feature of autonomy and socio-economic utility, especially for an information age, with evidence of age-related cognitive decline, add to a sense of bodily betrayal leaving persons vulnerable, risking further removal from the world. Such experience of senescence is disconcerting because it is a 'challenge to our relatively disembodied concerns and projects; and [opposing anthropological orthodoxies] it does so in circumstances not of our own choosing'.[68] Thus, experiences of loss and fears of further forfeiture begin to take effect. For the ageing, experiences of agency are constrained by finitude while capacities once thought basic recede into memory or become conditioned by a despairing dialectic of desire and fear.

Such images and experiences bristle against the icons of a modern subjectivity, disciplined to prioritize objective functions that can be tallied and tailored. This is reflected in the self-confidence of late modern humanity not only to strive for but also to secure control over the world, including ourselves according to our desires, by way of reason and technique. The anthropocentric confidence, however, is destabilized by frailty and finitude. The forerunners of death, whether disease or decay, are jolting to many; self-sufficiency, self-confidence and strength, vital competencies of a desiring agent, are confounded by the arresting dependencies which older age introduces and, at times, obliges.

Constrained, therefore, to rest in time rather than to revel in the world, as Améry depicts in his *On Ageing*, older persons are introduced to a reality, which encumbers independence and challenges functional depictions of dignity and meaningfulness. Confronted as such, many are set towards a despair, as described earlier.

Ageing, it seems, brings to the foreground both desire and fear. Ageing bodies, encumbered by unfettered discomforts and recurrent aches, revealing both frailty and finitude, bring to mind the accumulation of possessions, or desired functions, as well as the fear of losing them without expectations for their return – exciting anguish through which persons despair. Yet often with uncritical usage, or clarified delimitation, ageing persons are confronted with the promotion of *independence* as an ideal function for growing old successfully, which is, as noted above, a commonly cited principle and policy aim. As Chih Hoong Sin comments, discussions in ageing research, especially those where successful ageing, ageing well and healthy ageing is prioritized, often retain independence in later life as a value to secure.[69] Meanwhile, its opposite, dependence, retains a stigma and resources justifications for rationing the provision of services in accordance with economic demands.[70]

As Debbie Plath clarifies, with positive connotation, independence in the United Kingdom, is 'associated with pride in the ability to manage alone and control one's own life in older age'.[71] It is a concept closely associated with 'increased [consumer] choice and control by older people'.[72] Independence is presented as a policy that answers the problems of an ageing society and concerns over the 'situation of service dependency among older people that has developed in the past'.[73] Such policy inclusion does not disregard necessarily more nuanced concepts of independence that are socially inclusive, but the enduring and correlating concepts of 'freedom versus control; of autonomy and respect; and of dignity and choice;' do persist; such concepts 'do not chime well', as Sarah-Jane Fenton has commented, 'with notions of need for support and enablement'[74] – they do not chime well with those for whom the ideals of successful ageing are but fodder for despair; or, as Ina Jaffe stated despairingly in a NPR *Morning Edition* segment concerning phrases such as 'successful ageing', of which independence is a well-trod marker of achievement: 'I think it just means there's one more opportunity for me to fail'.[75]

The ideal of independence and the spectre of dependence haunts the third age, within which, in our late modern society, ageing persons are nurtured by images and icons of independence. The ideal of independence is captured by self-sufficiency, self-reliance and not being a burden. Such individualist and functional independence plagues many in the West as they grow ever older, as many are compelled by the depredations of ageing to consider themselves now in terms of dusk rather than dawn. Persons who have learned to understand independence as an individualistic ideal, tied to functional capacities, with positive notions of freedom of choice and of autonomy, confront the tyranny of an ageing body, paradoxically, where dependence is demanded.

Yet, drawing from Emil Cioran once again, '[W]e want to force the past, we want to act retroactively, to protest against the irreversible'.[76] Thus, in a concert of regret and despair, many persons, both older and younger, learn to lament dependence, to fear being cared for and to see the *mass of time* as a burden unsuited to human flourishing. Thus, persons in the late modern West learn to confront their experiences of ageing remembering past (desired) competencies (and fearing further loss) while abiding late modern ideals and in step with policy.

And, to be sure, many do press on. Pressing on for some, however, is as a repetition of late modern ideals that consider everything to be a mere 'contingent limitation'[77] that can be remediated and resolved. Such repetition nurtures a growing perspective, as American theologian Brent Waters has observed, that the body is also a mere remediable problem:

> an unwanted constraint against the will, and medicine should be dedicated to overcoming the limits of being embodied. Physicians are not expected to help patients to manage and come to terms with their finitude and mortality, but to wage an incessant war against these constraints with a growing arsenal of sophisticated technological weapons. The body should be an artifact of medical and technological ingenuity instead of an arbitrary given. The body, in short, is a problem to be solved.[78]

Yet such thinking does not reduce the risk for despair – rather, it heightens it. And for many ageing persons, they remain vulnerable to a despair which can overwhelm with its 'subjective torment'.[79] Such despair provokes these persons confronting the actualities of later life, according to the ideals of the late modern agency, to decide to control further that *problematic* life which becomes a life no longer worth living.

Pursuing Successes, Fearing Reality, Risking Despair

Reflecting on old age, at 97-year-old, philosopher Herbert Fingarette discusses the contra-rational exercise of pursuing successes that are oriented by memories of previously experienced abilities. Fingarette says, in the documentary *Being 97*, directed by his grandson Andrew Hasse,

> It is a loss of ability that you have had all your life. And there's a tendency to act as if you still had it and then fail, or be embarrassed. Or you have to accept that finally that you can't do that anymore. That's the rational thing to do. And it would be very nice if we just all did the rational thing to do. But we don't.[80]

Of course, for Fingarette, that we don't accept that which is reasonable, attending to the actualities of corporeality, makes sense: the abilities we once exercised 'are lifeline habits'.[81] Coming to terms with reality, especially with the need for special help from others, is a challenge for persons previously habituated by the performance of independence (and overcommitted to the problematic life). Yet reality can be, and often is, haunting.

Haunted by the fourth age, a predominant anthropology of the broken world constructs frail later life as a problem which ought to be disciplined or dispatched. The fourth age, for some, is as a kind of villain that threatens oppression and makes of life a misery. Accordingly, it is thought that such a life, such a villain, must be restrained ('as if burglars have to be fended off day and night'[82]). The disposition 'independence' and other such related priorities is a disposition that intends for persons to pursue absolute agency heroically, as though Heracles, who was able to overcome ageing.

Heracles, of course, is seen on an ancient artefact (a red-figure vase painting[83]) confronting Geras, the daemon or personification of Old Age.[84] Successful ageing strategies seem to invite ageing persons to do something similar. Such Heraclean agency, if I'm permitted to draw the allusion, essentializes independence in policy, where persons learn also to pursue the reified and abstracted imagery of older life that is frail and dependent as unwanted and catastrophic. Unwanted as a problem to overcome, successful ageing strategies with preoccupations of functional independence, in part, seem to point towards icons of human agency that mirror the Greek hero, who can master such a daemon of nature. After all, as the vase image depicts, it is Heracles whose posture exemplifies strength and vigour, or protest and resolve. Geras, the son of Nyx (Night), is depicted with his bent and emaciated body, 'a diminutive and repulsive figure'.[85] Without narrative (the mythical stories of Heracles and Geras have not survived) the red-figure vase imagery depicts Heracles not only pursuing but also threatening Geras with club in hand, to overcome the divinity of old age. So too are we all, invited as we are by policy and commodity and informed by a familiar academic model of 'successful ageing', to master the third age and to overcome the problem of the fourth age in later life. It is, after all, the principal message of John Rowe and Robert Kahn's model: 'successful ageing *is in our own hands*'.[86]

It is in our own hands to *compress* the experiences of morbidity and to achieve the functional ideals of the third age. Of course, 'compression of morbidity'[87] refers to the reduction in duration of chronic illness experienced at the end of life. Death, ideally, would be experienced suddenly or after a highly abbreviated duration of ailment that leads to death. My mother's stroke and death would serve as a quintessential example – the ideal that also suits the chronometric aspiration of Emanuel, who anticipates the *right* age to die.

Regarding 'compression of morbidity', as the authors of the forthcoming *Report of the Lancet Commission on the Value of Death*[88] make clear, advocates argue that chronic disease can be delayed by adapting one's lifestyle to accommodate more and more healthy or health-producing behaviours. Since it *can* be delayed, the moral argument follows that it *should* be delayed, driving the uptick in medical research and treatment interventions that correspond to the proposed ideal of morbidity.[89] But the responsibility to achieve such a compression, as successful ageing strategies and corresponding policies make clear, is ours, individually.

The relocation of ageing care from the responsibility of communities, including families and the professional societies elevated for special service, including health and medical personnel and related provisions, to the independent individual is indicative of late modern anthropology and technocratic social imaginaries.[90] Such imaginaries discipline a way of understanding individual and social life as a loose collection of 'responsible' independents who must, by their own functions plan and work for successes, whatever they might be. When considering ageing, *success* is dependent upon the individual to attain *it* through the functions of 'individual choice and effort'.[91] The continued administration and application of choice and effort by individuals is the hallmark of successful ageing imaginaries and requires the continuation of independent agency or productivity.[92]

'The onus is on the individual' to age well, successfully:[93] 'Just keep on going',[94] by choosing for yourself and by yourself to pursue fitness, healthfulness and happiness. Such pursuit is the journey of the hero, which promises the possibilities of building for oneself a better life.[95] Such imagery might seem fitting and 'hopeful'. That one can, by will, attain a better life or, by the administration of individual choice and independent effort, actively maintain the capacities for choice and effort throughout the life course and defeat the problem, Geras, is a repetition of the hero's journey.

But reality is not a Greek myth. And as I said above, such imagery is conjured and encouraged with risk. Such heroic imagery that elevates the individual to labour independently, as a responsibility of the good citizen (successful agent or responsible consumer or whatever the nomenclature), risks occluding one's vision to look carefully and honestly at corporeality and the actualities of later life. Such imagery does little to acknowledge that the Fourth age is not marked by chronometric time, as Jan Baars has critiqued.[96] It is marked, rather, by diminishing capacities, incumbent aches and the various losses persons experience as finite bodies (and bodies in relation to others) – losses like 'health, mobility, social status and social support', among others.[97]

The narrative tale we are told (and that we repeat to ourselves often), disciplined by a late modern anthropology, preoccupied with independence, for example, is that these capacities, aches and losses are ours alone to give an accounting. That is to say, should a person age poorly, unsuccessfully, such old age is the fault of no one except the individual who has failed to make good choices and productive effort – so, whatever that one is to do, she ought not to burden another for such malfeasance. Such 'failure' offers up the reason for one's experiences of frailty and dependence – leaving the person alone, responsible for her own fate.

In danger of such fate, of becoming *old*, we are told to press on and to labour diligently to remain young – choose youthfulness at every turn. It, youthfulness (viz. success), is, it seems, as any other commodity available by way of choice and diligent effort.[98] The paradigm of successful ageing is thus summarised as such: You too can be free from disease and disability, can maintain all physical capabilities, including cognitive capacity, and engage in life actively *if you decide*[99] – and we have all the measures and tools available to clarify and quantify where and how and when success has been achieved (or not).

Persons convinced by such a paradigm and conformed by the icons of the heroic will, shaped by a late modern anthropology, hold out for ideals, like perpetual independence, to be actualized. But when the creaking and crepitus begin to make noises anyway, when disease and dysfunction make heavy the labours of our daily activities, and our immanent exhaustion suspends our desires, we are set up for despair and schooled by fear, left without any narrative structure or perspective to help journey towards and through later life that makes the so-called problems of old age existentially *liveable* – 'independence', that is, as an ideal held up against the actualities of corporeality, reveals itself as nothing but fodder for our experiences of failure and a despair it nurtures.

Despairing of later life, we must also confront death. 'It's a frightening thought'![100]

Notes

1 Cioran, *Short History of Decay*, 96.

2 Ibid.

3 Valery Chirkov, et al., 'Differentiating autonomy from individualism and independence: A self-determination theory perspective on internalization of cultural orientations and well-being', *Journal of Personality and Social Psychology* 84, no. 1 (2003): 97–110 (98).

4 Giddens, *Modernity and Self-Identity*, 213.

5 Laura M. Ahearn, 'Language and agency', *Annual Review of Anthropology* 30 (2001): 109–137.

6 Chris Gilleard and Paul Higgs, 'Aging without agency: Theorizing the fourth age', *Aging & Mental Health* 14, no. 2 (2010): 121–128.

7 Diego Romaioli and Alberta Contarello, 'Redefining agency in late life: The concept of "disponibility"', *Ageing and Society* 39, no. 1 (2019): 194–216 (212n1). Emphasis is mine.

8 Debbie Plath, 'Independence in old age: The route to social exclusion?', *British Journal of Social Work* 38, no. 7 (2008): 1353–1369.

9 Elena Portacolone, 'The myth of independence for older Americans living alone in the Bay Area of San Francisco: A critical reflection', *Ageing and Society* 31, no. 5 (2011): 803–828 (815).

10 Ian Mortimer, 'The Triumph of the Doctors: Medical Assistance to the Dying, C. 1570–1720 (The Alexander Prize Essay)', *Transactions of the Royal Historical Society* 15 (2005): 97–116 (116).

11 Zahava Gabriel and Ann Bowling, 'Quality of life from the perspectives of older people', *Ageing and Society* 24, no. 5 (2004): 675–691; Susan Tester, et al., 'Frailty and institutional life', in *Growing Older. Quality of Life in Old Age*, eds. Alan Walker and Catherin Hagan Hennessy (Maidenhead: Open University Press, 2004), 209–224.

12 Plath, 'Independence in Old Age', 1353–1369.

13 Fiona Robinson, 'Resisting hierarchies through relationality in the ethics of care', *International Journal of Care and Caring* 4, no. 1 (2020): 11–23.

14 James Stark, *The Cult of Youth: Anti-ageing in Modern Britain* (Cambridge: Cambridge University Press, 2020).

15 Marcel, *Homo Viator*, 36.

16 Ibid.

17 Anne P. F. Wand, et al., 'Why do the very old self-harm? A qualitative study', *American Journal of Geriatric Psychiatry* 26, no. 8 (2018): 862–871 (866).

18 Marcel, *Homo Viator*, 47.

19 Peter Laslett, 'The emergence of the third age', *Ageing and Society* 7, no. 2 (1987): 133–160. For further discussion of the 'fourth age imaginary', see Chris Gilleard and Paul Higgs, 'Ageing without agency: Theorizing the fourth age', *Ageing and Mental Health* 14, no. 2 (2010): 121–128; Paul Higgs and Chris Gilleard, *Rethinking Old Age: Theorising the Fourth Age* (London: Palgrave Macmillan, 2015).

20 Richard M. Suzman, David P. Willis and Kenneth Manton, eds., *The Oldest Old* (Oxford: Oxford University Press, 1992).

21 See Peter Laslett, 'The emergence of the third age', *Ageing and Society* 7, no. 2 (1987): 133–160; Peter Laslett, *A Fresh Map of Life: The Emergence of the Third Age* (Cambridge: Harvard University Press, 1991).

22 Sørensen, 'The paradox of modern suffering', 141.

23 Améry, *On Ageing*.

24 Anne Case and Angus Deaton, 'Rising midlife morbidity and mortality, US whites', *Proceedings of the National Academy of Sciences* 112, no. 49 (2015): 15078–15083; Anne Case and Angus Deaton, *Deaths of Despair and the Future of Capitalism* (Princeton: Princeton University Press, 2020).

25 Paul Stenner, Tara McFarquhar and Ann Bowling, 'Older people and "active ageing": Subjective aspects of ageing actively', *Journal of Health Psychology* 16, no. 3 (2011): 467–477 (273).

26 Eileen M. Crimmins, 'Trends in the health of the elderly', *Annual Review of Public Health* 25, no. 1 (2004): 79–98; Kaare Christensen, et al., 'Ageing populations: The challenges ahead', *Lancet* 374, no. 9696 (2009): 1196–1208; and Robert F. Schoeni, Vicki A. Freedman and Linda G. Martin, 'Why is late-life disability declining?', *Milbank Quarterly* 86, no. 1 (2008): 48–89.

27 Sandra Torres and Gubhild Hammerström, 'Speaking of 'limitations' while trying to disregard them: A qualitative study of how diminished everyday competence and aging can be regarded', *Journal of Aging Studies* 20, no. 4 (2006): 291–302.

28 Loise Aronson, *Elderhood: Redefining Aging, Transforming Medicine, Reimagining Life* (New York: Bloomsbury, 2021), 317.

29 Jan Baars, *Aging and the Art of Living* (Baltimore: Johns Hopkins University Press, 2012), 205–206, 243–244.

30 Els van Wijngaarden, Carlo Leget and Anne Goossensen, 'Experiences and motivations underlying wishes to die in older people who are tired of living: A research area in its infancy', *OMEGA—Journal of Death and Dying* 69, no. 2 (2014): 191–216; '[Tiredness of life] (or weariness of life or life fatigue) is defined as suffering caused by the prospect of having to continue living with a very poor quality of life, not predominantly caused by a physical or psychiatric disease, and closely associated with a death wish' (Liesbeth van Humbeeck, et al., 'Tiredness of life in older persons: A qualitative study on nurses' experiences of being confronted with this growing phenomenon', *The Gerontologist* 60, no. 4 (2019): 735–744 (736).

31 Iris D. Hartog, et al., 'Prevalence and characteristics of older adults with a persistent death wish without severe illness: A large cross-sectional survey', *BMC Geriatrics* 20, no. 342 (2020): doi.org/10.1186/s12877-020-01735-0.

32 Van Wijngaarden, 'Experiences and motivations underlying wishes to die', 197.

33 Ibid., 202.

34 Els van Wijngaarden, Carlo Leget and Anne Goossensen, 'Ready to give up on life: The lived experience of elderly people who feel life is completed and no longer worth living', *Social Science and Medicine* 138 (2015): 257–264 (260).

35 Alison L. Chasteen, 'The role of age and age-related attitudes in perceptions of elderly individuals', *Basic and Applied Social Psychology* 22, no. 3 (2000): 147–156; Scott M. Lynch, 'Measurement and prediction of aging anxiety', *Research on Aging* 22, no. 5 (2000): 533–558; Becca R. Levy, 'Mind matters: Cognitive and physical effects of aging self-stereotypes', *The Journals of Gerontology: Series B* 58, no. 4 (2003): 203–211; Pnina Ron, 'Elderly people's attitudes and perceptions of aging and old age: The role of cognitive dissonance', *Geriatric Psychiatry* 22, no. 7 (2007): 656–622; and Rhonda Shaw and Matthew Langman, 'Perceptions of being old and the ageing process', *Ageing International* 42 (2017): 115–135.

36 Nietzsche, *Will to Power*, 22.

37 Ibid.
38 Van Wijngaarden, et al., 'Ready to give up on life', 260. Emphasis is mine.
39 Warnes, 'Being old', 298.
40 Ibid., 305.
41 Jane Aronson, '"I don't want to be a burden": Needing assistance in a context of disentitlement', *Canadian Woman Studies/Les Cahiers de la Femme* 12, no. 2 (1992): 65–67 (65). Emphasis is mine.
42 Ibid., 65.
43 Mari Lloyd-Williams, et al., 'The end of life: A qaulitative study of the perceptions of people over the age of 80 on issues surrounding death and dying', *Journal of Pain and Symptom Management* 34, no. 1 (2007): 60–66 (62).
44 Christine J. McPherson, Keith G. Wilson and Mary Ann Murray, 'Feeling like a burden: Exploring the perspectives of patients at the end of life', *Social Science & Medicine* 64, no. 2 (2007): 417–427 (418).
45 Danielle R. Jahn, Kimberley A. Van Orden and Kelly C. Cukrowicz, 'Perceived burdensomeness in older adults and perceptions of burden on spouses and children', *Clinical Gerontologicst* 36, no. 5 (2013): 451–459 (452).
46 McPherson, et al., 'Feeling like a burden', 423.
47 Ibid.
48 Ibid., 421.
49 Van Wijngaarden, et al., 'Experiences and motivations underlying wishes to die', 206; Van Wijngaarden, et al., 'Ready to give up on life', 260.
50 Andrea Charise, '"Let the reader think of the burden': Old age and the crisis of capacity', *Occasion: Interdisciplinary Studies in the Humanities* 4 (2012): 1–16 (3). Accessed July 2021. https://arcade.stanford.edu/sites/default/files/article_pdfs/OCCASION_v04_Charise_053112_0.pdf
51 Warnes, 'Being old', 329.
52 As quoted by Charise, 'Let the reader think of the burden', 1–2; cf. Amanda S. Barusch, 'The ageing tsunami: Time for a new metaphor?', *Journal of Gerontological Social Work* 56, no. 3 (2013): 181–184.
53 Warnes, 'Being old', 297–298.
54 Darcy McMaughan, Rachel Edwards and Bita Kash, 'The Methusian catastrophe', *Primary Health Care* 3, no. 2 (2013): 1–3.
55 Alan Walker, 'The economic "burden" of ageing and the prospect of intergenerational conflict', *Ageing & Society* 10, no. 4 (1990): 377–396 (378).
56 Aubrey deGrey and Michael Rae, *Ending Aging: The Rejuvenation Breakthrough That Could Reverse Human Aging in Our Lifetime* (New York: St. Martin, 2007).
57 Améry, *On Ageing*, 35.
58 Ibid., 20.
59 Emanuel, 'Why I hope to die at 75', para 25.
60 Améry, *On Ageing*, 46.
61 Louise Crocker, L. Clare and K. Evans, 'Giving up or finding a solution? The experience of attempted suicide in later life', *Aging & Mental Health* 10, no. 6 (2006): 638–647 (641).
62 Améry, *On Ageing*, 42.
63 Chris Gilleard and Paul Higgs, 'Unacknowledged distinctions: Corporeality versus embodiment in later life', *Journal of Aging Studies* 45 (2018): 5–10 (6).

64 Baars, *Ageing and the Art Living*, 243–244.

65 Améry, *On Ageing*, 34.

66 Kevin McKee and Marynn Gott, 'Shame and the ageing body', In *Body Shame: Conceptualization, Research, and Treatment*, eds. P. Gilbert and J. Miles (London: Routledge, 2002), 75–89.

67 Gilleard and Higgs, 'Unacknowledged distinctions', 8.

68 Ibid., 6.

69 Chih Hoong Sin, 'Older people from white-British and Asian-Indian backgrounds and their expectations for support from their children', *Quality in Ageing and Older Adults* 8, no. 1 (2007): 31–41.

70 Debbie Plath, 'International policy perspectives on independence in old age', *Journal of Aging & Social Policy* 21, no. 2 (2009): 209–223.

71 Ibid., 218.

72 Ibid.

73 Ibid.

74 Sarah-Jane Fenton, 'Ageing and agency: The contested gerontological landscape of control, security, and independence and the need for ongoing care and support', *Birmingham Policy Commission* (2014): 1–8 (3). Retrieved 3 September 2020. https://www.birmingham.ac.uk/Documents/research/policycommission/healthy-ageing/5-Ageing-and-agency-control-and-independence-updated.pdf

75 Ina Jaffee and NPR Staff, '"Silver Tsunami" and other terms that can irk the over-65 set', *Morning Edition* (Radio broadcast): NPR (14 May 2014). https://www.npr.org/2014/05/19/313133555/silver-tsunami-and-other-terms-that-can-irk-the-over-65-set

76 Cioran, *Short History of Decay*, 32.

77 Baars, *Ageing and the Art of Living*, 243.

78 Brent Waters, 'Technology, distractions, and the care of the body', *Human Flourishing Blog* (October 2019), para. 4. Retrieved 10 July 2020. https://www.patheos.com/blogs/humanflourishing/2019/10/technology-distractions-and-the-care-of-the-body/

79 Cioran, *Short History of Decay*, 37.

80 From Andrew Hasse's documentary 'Being 97': Herbert Fingarette and Andrew Hasse, 'A 97-year-old philosopher faces his own death: "What is the point?" | The Atlantic', Online video clip. *The Atlantic*, 18:12 (14 January 2020). https://www.theatlantic.com/video/index/604840/being-97/ (2:32–3:15).

81 Fingarette, 'Being 97', 3:36.

82 Baars, *Aging and the Art of Living*, 69.

83 Heracles and Geras, Red-Figure Vase Painting (Louvre G234), Musée du Louvre, Paris (Beazley Archive No. 202622).

84 Cecil Smith, 'Vase with representation of Herakles and Geras', *The Journal of Hellenic Studies* 4 (1883): 96–110.

85 Smith, 'Vase with Herakles and Geras', 105.

86 John W. Rowe and Robert L. Kahn, *Successful Aging* (New York: Pantheon, 1998), 18. Emphasis is mine.

87 Introduced by James Fries, 'Aging, natural death, and the compression of morbidity', *New England Journal of Medicine* 303 (1980): 130–135.

88 I am making reference here to an unpublished draft of the forthcoming *Report of the Lancet Commission on the Value of Death*. However, the initial discussion regarding 'compression of morbidity' has been included at The Value of Death web blog: Seamus O'Mahony, 'The compression of morbidity: A real phenomenon or just wishful thinking?', *The Value of Death*, (19 September 2019). https://commissiononthevalueofdeath.wordpress.com/2019/09/19/the-compression-of-morbidity-a-real-phenomenon-or-just-wishful-thinking/

89 Even when evidence does not support the argument that favors compression of morbidity: prevalence of chronic disease is likely to increase rather than decrease, resulting in an 'expansion, no compression, of morbidity' (Andrew Kingston, et al., 'Projections of multi-morbidity in the older population in England to 2035: estimates from the Population Ageing and Care Simulation (PACSim) model', *Age Ageing* 47, no. 3 (2018): 374–380). For some, compression of morbidity is as fodder for illusions of immortality; yet the concept continues to hold prominence (Eileen M. Crimmins and Hiram Beltrán-Sánchez, 'Mortality and morbidity trends: Is there compression of morbidity?', *Journal of Gerontology: Social Sciences. Series B, Psychological Sciences and Social Sciences* 66, no. 1 (2011): 75–86).

90 See Carol J. Greenhouse, *Ethnographies of Neoliberalism* (Philadelphia: University of Pennsylvania Press, 2010).

91 Rowe and Kahn, *Successful Aging*, 37.

92 Robert L. Rubinstein and Kate de Medeiros, '"Successful aging", gerontological theory and neoliberalism: A qualitative critique', *The Gerontologist* 55, no. 1 (2015): 43–42 (38–39).

93 Ibid., 36.

94 Rowe and Kahn, *Successful Aging*, 40; cf. Rubinstein and deMederos, 'Successful Ageing', 39.

95 Mary Godfrey, Jean Townsend and Tracy Denby, *Building a Good Life for Older People in Local Communities: The Experience of Ageing in Time and Place* (York: Joseph Rowntree Foundation, 2004), 2.

96 '[C]hronometric age is an over-rated and rather superficial way to generalize across individuals who are very different [...] in terms of their functional capacities' (Baars, *Aging and Art of Living*, 68).

97 Crocker, et al., 'Giving up or finding a solution', 643.

98 Baars, *Aging and Art of Living*, 66–74.

99 Rowe and Kahn, *Successful Aging*, 433. Emphasis is mine.

100 Fingarette, 'Being 97', 14:03.

Chapter 3

DYING DECEIVED BY DESPAIR
IN DISGUISE

'I am going to die'.
'I am going to die on my own terms'.

These two statements stand as resolute declarations, which persons might pronounce about their dying. However, the two statements are not equivalent.

With the former, 'I am going to die', I am reminded of the words a terminal cancer patient shared with me many years ago while I was working at a cancer clinic and researching chemotherapy-induced peripheral neuropathies.[1] Patricia refused all further treatments and was explicit about her readiness to die. She was an ailing woman with an aggressive pancreatic cancer and metastatic disease, suffering significant fatigue and numbness, tingling and pain in her limbs from previous treatment rounds. Her body was gauntly, her skin a pale palate of whites and reds, and her eyes set paradoxically tired and alert on her face. She was confronting the imminent threat of death. Yet, her living towards the *mystery*[2] of life inclusive of death while revealing the fullness of her frailties and dependencies seemed to consider death as an end in itself. While I cannot say that she *wanted* to live as such (as an expression of pure will), she certainly did live knowing she was in the midst of death. She lived opposing the familiar logic of several oncologists I had come to know who always seemed to have another treatment available.

Her cancer, although differing in origin, was similar to that of journalist A. A. (Adrian Anthony) Gill who, at 62, described his metastatic lung cancer as 'an embarrassment of cancer, the full English'.[3] He would go on to describe, 'There is barely a morsel of offal not included'. The oncologist who was treating Gill, predictably it seems, 'dangled before this dying man a drug that he knew he couldn't prescribe […] [and] which give very modest survival gains in most […] but are presented to the patient as a sure thing'.[4] Gill penned an essay for *The Times* (appearing 11 December 2016), through which he begrudged the NHS for not paying out so that patients might procure such treatments

(Hope can be contemptuous). Patricia too was offered similar, experimental interventions – she refused these with certain realism: 'I am going to die'.

With the latter, 'I am going to die on my own terms', I am reminded of Simon Critchley's claim that 'Death is not usually chosen as an end in itself, but for some other reason'.[5] As he suggests, some people choose to die in order to avoid pain and suffering while others choose to die for a cause. Perhaps one can choose to die because of both reasons: the suicide note of Charlotte Perkins Gilman, who was 75 years old, might suggest that she chose to die in order to avoid the depredations of cancer *and* to offer her death as a message that might challenge previously held social convictions: 'Believing this choice to be of social service in promoting wiser view on this question, I have preferred Chloroform to cancer'.[6] Hers was to be regarded an election for death in order to achieve other ends (at very least to foreswear a natural, viz. uncontrolled, death, whatever that might mean in an already highly medicalized milieu).

Consequently, 'I am going to die on my own terms' reminds me of the non-profit Death with Dignity [USA] National Center, which states that 'the greatest human freedom is to live, and die, according to one's own desires and beliefs'.[7] Death with Dignity's aim to secure such freedom is an objective shared by others, like Jo Roman. Her belief that suicide can be rational (thus freely chosen) and not simply pathological is read, for example, in her suicide note, which also reveals (all-caps included) her desire to die free from unwanted distresses: 'By the time you read these lines I WILL HAVE GENTLY ENDED my life on the date of this letter's postmark. [...] I decided I would set an exit date and prepare to meet it. I'd aim for my exit date to predate discomfort of intensity which might diminish my chance of CREATING ON MY OWN TERMS THE FINAL STROKE OF MY LIFE'S CANVAS'.[8]

The latter statement reflects an increasingly prevalent disposition that persons ought to be permitted to die as they desire – with the onus to age well independently (as one acts and chooses for herself) remains the onus to die well too. That is to suggest, persons ought to be given the freedom to die as a practice of choice and a progress (or achievement) in moral technique. Such deaths, like the functions of independence, the rhetoric infers, preserve 'dignity'.

Dignity here is conditional upon self-determination, or the execution of choice free from coercive influences, including untamed experiences incumbent to frailty and disease. Dignity is thus functional too, connected to a particular rational decision that is regarded as congruent with one's beliefs and values (viz. desires). That is to say, for those who desire a 'good death', meaning a death coordinated to one's beliefs and values, society should establish the legal and medical provisions to ensure persons are not obligated to face the inescapable and terrifying fate of the human condition.[9] The good death might be likened here to the 'nice trip'[10] that one chooses to take in order to find respite from the grind of daily life. In the case of those confronting irremediable disease and unrelenting suffering, the 'trip', however, is permanent – and, ultimately, annihilates one's freedom for such *wise* decision.[11]

Nevertheless, the positive act of 'Death with Dignity', or medical assistance in dying (MAiD), is narrated as a (rightful) freedom that ought to be respected by others and made legally available for persons who desire to self-govern the experiences and expressions of their living and dying. It is narrated as the way to secure a freedom, to liberate oneself, from experiences of anguish and despair – whether experienced presently or forecasted as an eventual future.

It offers a kind of hopeful *optimism* for relief from a human condition many fear – a condition marked, as we read previously, by disease, decay, depredation and dependency. Of course, few would argue hope is needed for persons confronting such limits of human life, which are antagonised not only by the threats of death but also the pains and sufferings that correspond to human corporeality. Yet, as we are doing in this book, one must discriminate of what kind of hope one is pursuing and/or discovering. After all, despair can masquerade as hope. Put differently, the illusion of hope can, in fact, be a delusion.[12]

The following, therefore, will extend the argument which began previously, studying the vulnerability to despair that accompanies our growing older in our late modern age. Giving attention to particular expressions of autonomy, which persist as fodder for despair in our late modern milieu, the late classical account of Heracles and his death, as well as contemporary reasons for soliciting medical assistance in dying, will focus the discrimination of despair as hope in disguise – a despair that anticipates voluntary dying, whether by one's own hand or by MAiD. I first orient us to the prevalence of autonomy in the late modern imagination. Its triumph is marked by the commonplace pre-eminence of the doctrine, which correlates individual freedom (and dignity) with the Heraclean capacity to determine for oneself all matters of rational concern (i.e. to resolve one's problems). It is by way of one's rational agency (viz. autonomy), protected by the respect for one's autonomy by others, that hope is discussed. Hope remains for those persons who are able to exercise rational agency free from coercive influence – one can remain hopeful if they are able to execute on the freedom to make rational choices (to elect for what they want or against what they do not want).

So, it might be that MAiD offers hope for the hopeless – those persons whose diagnoses are irremediable and whose sufferings are unremitting.

Some might suggest, for example, that MAiD, whether by physician assistance or active administration, offers hope for a good death, which is conditioned by *freedoms* to elect for the timing and conditions by which one might die. That freedom is thought essential for the late modern subject and it is the prognoses of disease that demand the exercise of such liberty. Such freedom, delimited by unencumbered choice, confers hope, so it is thought.

While it might be a 'hope', it is of a very particular and, ultimately, corrupt kind. Concluding that such an understanding of hope leaves persons vulnerable to experience despair, the chapter turns to demonstrate the ways in which a modern anthropology that conditions us to believe in the preeminence of autonomy occludes or overshadows the actualities of despair; and persons are thus given over to it. People risk becoming incapable of seeing they both loathe and idolize the life conjured and concretized by a late modern imagination. Thus, finally, illuminating the patterns or practices of hopelessness, I show where and how persons confronting the depredations of corporeality, decay and disease, both physical and psychological, as well as persons dutifully charged to give care to such persons, are deceived by hope masquerading as despair. Such a masquerade allows persons to die in (even from) despair but with only illusions of control (autonomy) persisting and without realistic hope at all.

Triumph of Autonomy, Conferring Hope

MAiD is argued by advocates and apologists to be both a 'triumph of autonomy' and consistent with the 'traditional commitment' of the physician towards the patient.[13] By autonomy, triumph refers to the liberty of patients to determine their lives and deaths by the administration of one's rational agency that is free from coercive influence. Traditional commitment refers to the competent clinical practice and rational care for those confronting pain, suffering and the threats of death. Now, one should note, the 'traditional' commitment is arguably quite novel. Emerging with the seventeenth century Age of Reason (Enlightenment) and in the wake of the Renaissance, physicians and surgeons referred to with elevated status as 'doctors' (*docero*, teacher) convinced the ill, infirmed and dying that they had increased choice to elect for rational care of, perhaps over, their lives – enabling individuals to take responsibility for themselves.[14] They were not merely cornered by fate or determined by fear-filled patience for divine action, but convinced they could possess the world of their desires (and relieved of their fears). Thus, the medicine of the day and the determinative attention to disease provided by the doctors offered option for control over the 'landscape of disease' wherein such medical practice and prescription bolstered a medical individualism, or agency, that continues, arguably triumphs, in our current milieu. Such control over disease is, in fact, regarded as 'a very special thing', when applied to 'a self-willed ending', as Bert Keizer a physician affiliated with the *Expertisecentrum Euthanasie* (Expertise Centre Euthanasia) in the Netherlands expressed in *The Guardian*.[15] Thus, as such a triumph of autonomy, MAiD signals for many a significant achievement of concrete, self-conscious agency; the strong modern subject capable to master fate by electing for the good death.

The ideal subject is thus the one who is enabled to recognize the problems of living in this world and who possesses the reason and will to do-against-death and to control destiny. Perhaps this is why *health* is argued to be a prototypical value – it is by health (biomedically understood as one's physical, mental and social competence) an individual is viewed by self and others as capable to guarantee her self-actualization, achieving what is essential and meaningful to her.[16] Both hospice and medical assistance in dying draw upon such a familiar script, suggesting the modern agent ought to be free to have a death that accords with her own terms (her desires and fears), thus preserving the essential self and producing the good death.[17] Thus, whether sustaining the pursuit of self for as long as possible until biological death takes hold (akin to compression of morbidity, for example) or bringing death to the foreground in order to avoid the risk of losing one's self prematurely (as in cases of dementia, for example), the imagery of self-sufficiency and individual faculty is apropos.

Yet, the mechanics of modern medicine aim towards similar ends – towards such self-actualization – to the extent that reason and will could be regarded as chief values of the medical institution and the professionals it forms in our late modern Western society. It is by way of health, by the administration of will and reason in our physical, mental and social lives, that medicine and its providers can serve its constituents. Medicine can help to produce the *thing*, that is, health, persons want to have.

After all, as the WHO congress gave assent, 'Health is no longer an optional matter, but the golden key to the relief of human misery. We must be well'.[18] Without *it*, as the logic concludes, life is miserable. Thus, we must exercise absolute agency in matters of life and death. The heroic archetype, who is poised to exercise agency-as-might, must also exercise justice as he sets out 'in search of monsters to slay, crimes to avenge, [and] deep-seated wrongs to right'.[19] And, as the politics of MAiD contend, there are few greater wrongs to right (or problems to resolve) than irremediable disease (for some, this includes ageing) and unrelenting agony.

Vivian Sleight argues thusly: 'To have the option to choose voluntary euthanasia confers hope—the hope of a good death'.[20] For Sleight, such hope is conditioned by the ideation that a good death can be secured by the administration of choice (informed consent) and the respect of medical professionals and legal authorities to abide such choice (respect for autonomy). Such hope functions as a sort of optimism where we not only imagine our future but also recognize our past, aiming to secure those values or ideals we have and thought essential. For the patient, MAiD confers 'hope of control, resurgence of identity, and personal dignity'.[21] For the physician, MAiD secures their intention to rehearse the traditional commitments of medical practice and 'to relieve suffering'.[22]

However, such a hope might be thought as a functional hoping. Such hope might be categorized as an objective hope caught up into a technological rationality, which aims to secure, by the administration of procedure, policy, or programme, the delimited values one desires (or fears will be lost). Such hope is to be given or received by the administration of one's agency and the cooperative agency of others intending to respect autonomy, in pursuit of such aims. This type of hoping might be exemplified by the phrase that 'I hope that [*fill in the blank*] will happen'. For Sleight, one might fill in the blank with, 'I hope that *a good death* will happen'. Alternatively, the phrasing might be given as above: 'I hope that *I can die on my own terms*'. Or 'I hope that *I can die by MAiD*' before I experience insufferable depredations of frailty and advanced disease – especially before dementia removes the possibilities to exercise agency at will (to be eligible for MAiD services in most jurisdictions where assisted dying is permissible).

Reciprocally, then, the good death pursued by modern agency is thought only to be secured by the actualization of such agency. Linking the logic of patient-directed refusals of treatment when such treatments are futile with the petition for assisted dying, Sleight offers up a narrative that champions the sort of thinking, which autonomy has proffered in contemporary late modern bioethics while suggesting such thinking procures or produces the hope. The kind of hope Sleight has in mind is bolstered further by claims and legislations that secure the individual's right for such a commodity.

Such hoping, however, is but as a masquerade. The logic of such functional hoping to procure a given, concrete, end (an ideal or commodity or desire, for example) is but fodder for despair. It is hope corrupted. One need only to raise the following questions to begin the interrogation of such hopes:

What happens when our values go unfulfilled? What happens when such aims prove aimless and the mechanics of desire show their frailty and their limit? What happens when health cannot be achieved? What happens when the individual places her trust in the institution of medicine, (only) to discover that it cannot secure on her behalf either freedom or happiness against the limits of physical, mental and social dis-ease? What happens when

Heracles (the one who was introduced as an icon of human agency, committed to overthrow ageing, is now taken by 'a strange disease [that he] [...] cannot withstand by courage, weapons, or strength'.[23]

These questions are relevant to the contemporary turn towards MAiD. The concrete experiences of both patients at the end of life and their physicians, among other health professionals and carers, serve as the ground from which the questions above arise – questions that require further reflection.

The Triumph of Autonomy, Occluding Despair

As was illumined above, autonomy has become a principal doctrine that delimits and defines the human subject in late modernity. Self-determination is anthropological orthodoxy – a function of having a will free from coercive influence, which we desire to maintain and fear losing. For medicine, this has meant the increased role for patients in electing for medical care. The subsequent attention given by medical professionals aims not only to respect patient autonomy but also to facilitate the *free* choices (desires) of patients. That free choice has extended to petitions for increased control over the timing and circumstances of one's dying in order to achieve the good, viz. self-willed and controlled, death. Yet the conclusion raised questions about such functional hoping, the way 'hope' works for many persons confronting death. In fact, I have already suggested that such hopes are corrupt; mere *fodder for despair*. The following shows this to be the case – the triumph of autonomy in modern bioethics, and the pre-eminence of an incumbent Heraclean anthropology, not only risks but also occludes despair, while also allowing persons, so it is argued, to escape their present or pending experiences of life amidst death. However, such escape is not due to an exercise of free rational agency, due to the triumph of autonomy, but by way of the fear and anxiety, that is, the despair, that persists.

We shall begin with the reasons persons elect for MAiD: The reasons given, as you might imagine, are numerous. Yet reporting is often general. The annual reporting, or press releases, from the *Commission fédérale de Contrôle et d'Évaluation de l'Euthanasie* includes a general description that the majority of persons soliciting MAiD suffer from both physical *and* psychological suffering (84.6% of 2444 persons in Belgium, 2020), with the remaining individuals suffering from either physical or psychological suffering.[24] Yet, the nature of the suffering is not further delimited and the reasons patients might reveal to physicians not included. This is similar in the annual report from Luxembourg's *Commission Nationale de Contrôle et d'Évaluation de l'application de la loi du 16 mars 2009 sur l'euthanasie et l'assistance au suicide*, which briefly summarizes the nature of suffering experienced – reporting, briefly, the suffering has all been described as constant, unbearable and without expectation for improvement.[25]

That said, annual reports from Oregon, Washington and Canada, for example, offer more exacting details, reporting a range of specific (and often combined) reasons persons might solicit MAiD. Oregon's *Death with Dignity Act* relative statistics (2020 [and total, since 1998]), for example, reveal poor pain control, or concern about it, (32.7 [27.4%]) and prohibitive costs of treatment (6.1% [4.5%]) are considered as less significant reasons than other concerns. Loss of autonomy and control over bodily functions (93.1% and 39.8% [90.6% and 43.1%], respectively), reduced participation in daily activities that make life enjoyable (94.3% [89.9%]), perceived or threatened loss of dignity (71.8% [73.6%]) and sensitivity of becoming a burden for others (53.1% [47.5%]) are assessed as the principal reasons for soliciting MAiD.[26] Similarly, the *Washington State Death with Dignity Act Report* suggests loss of autonomy (90%) and bodily control (46%), diminished activities of daily life (87%), loss of dignity (73%) and risk of being a burden (56%) persist as principal concerns that motivate decisions to elect for MAiD.[27] Hence, whether one can observe these losses immediately or at some future state of impairment, such reasons do yield sufficient cause for patients to die, as they might say, on their own terms, with dignity intact.

Similar reporting is seen in the Second Annual Report on MAiD in Canada.[28] Eligibility for MAiD in Canada is determined, in part, on patient experiences of severe, intolerable suffering, provoked by a grievous and irremediable medical condition, whether physical or psychological. Accordingly, medical personnel, including physicians and nurse practitioners for example, are required to solicit and to report on how persons might describe the nature of their suffering – with losses in the ability to participate in meaningful activities and in the ability to perform activities of daily living cited most frequently (at 84.9% and 81.7% of the 7,384 MAiD death reports received by Health Canada). Similar to the reporting above, 35.9% or 2,650 individuals reported self-perceived burden as a contributing factor of their suffering. Loss of dignity was also a significant factor for 53.9% of persons soliciting MAiD. However, unlike reporting from Washington and Oregon, inadequate (concern over) control of pain was quite frequently reported, at 53.9%.

In addition to these statistics coming from official reports, relevant literature that has surveyed patients requesting MAiD, along with carers and others offering support for MAiD, corroborates and clarifies the reasons given. For example, several studies have shown desire for control over the circumstances of death for patients seeking MAiD is considered important by proxies, including both medical and nursing professionals as well as ancillary service providers (i.e. hospice chaplains and social workers).[29] Moreover, those persons soliciting MAiD have also included as principal reasons the loss of independence, a desire to control the time and manner of death, the risk of becoming a burden and the prospect of worsening pain or quality of life.[30]

Robert Pearlman and his colleagues have also observed that persons are motivated to pursue MAiD due to a range of fears and losses, including but not limited to pain.[31] Diminished sense of self, yearnings to regain control and fear concerning possible future states of being, or simply death, alongside functional losses and persistent fatigue, contributed significantly to the rationale to pursue MAiD. Put differently, the failure to maintain or to secure the characteristics of autonomy has contributed significantly not only to the ideation but also the solicitation for medically mediated death.

These reasons are corroborated further by Maggie Hendry and her fellow researcher's systematic review of literature that asked the following: 'Why do we want the right to die?'. The study revealed the following in response to the question: factors such as feeling to be a burden, loss of interest or pleasure, loneliness and diminished quality of life and control contributed significantly to the reasons for wanting the right to die.[32] Although not associated with pain per se, in a biomedical sense, these reasons were tied to patient experiences and expressions of 'unbearable suffering' and reflect psycho-emotional, socio-environmental and existential vulnerabilities to despair. They reflect a succumbing to hopelessness, which additional findings echo.

For example, Marianne Dees and her colleagues observed 'all patients [interviewed] considered hopelessness to be a main factor in the perception of unbearableness'.[33] Dees and her colleagues listened to patients, who related statements as follows: An 80-year-old male declared, 'I can't do anything anymore, I used to play music, participated in various clubs, all so very companionable, I had to say farewell to all of it. It feels so awful just waiting to become bedridden and then waiting to die'.[34] A 50-year-old female lamented, 'You lie on a bed and none of the normal functions come back. They will never come back, and it will only get worse'.[35] Concomitantly, Martina Pestinger and her collaborators recorded similar sentiments concerning the theme of failed self-determination in the ideation to hasten death:

[Participant 11] They [relatives and caregivers] do not feel the agonies, but I do. Now it has come so far, that I am only lying here. You think. You think and think and you bring many things to mind and passing in revue I have come to a decision, yes, well [...] I am lying waiting for death.

[Participant 7] Activities with friends are not possible—and indeed activities outside or with the faculty, I would say, meanwhile completely pass away.

[Participant 2] This is a bit of a vicious circle. When my wife sees that I am doing badly then that makes her suffer. Then I see that my wife is suffering severely and then I—because I know that basically it is my fault. If you can talk about a fault.

[Participant 8] I am not used to somebody helping me. This I feel is tantalizing, this is no life.[36]

Similarly, and returning again to official reports, the *Regionale Toetsingscommissies Euthanasie* [Regional Euthanasia Review Committees] in The Netherlands has issued their *Jaarverslag* 2020 [Annual Report 2020] in which case studies reiterate, in one way or another, the statistically collated reasons offered above as well as the reported patient statements.[37] Case 2020-153, for example, introduces the reader to a woman between 70 and 80 years of age with ovarian cancer and with no surgical or effective treatment options available. Palliative measures to manage pain and discomfort also proved under-effective and the woman experienced suffering in various ways, including limited intake of food and hydration because of persistent nausea and fatigue. The experiences of fatigue encumbered previously enjoyed activities, including reading and viewing television. Losses of appetite and energy goaded fears of suffering from further losses of function. Accordingly, to the doctor, it was evident the woman 'was exhausted':

> The woman was known as a positive person who valued her quality of life. That such quality of life was now difficult to find, the doctor understood the suffering experienced by the woman had become unbearable. Moreover, because there was a severe ovarian cancer (grade 3c) diagnosis with metastases in the peritoneum (peritonitis carcinomatosa), and there was no way for the suffering to be alleviated, the doctor was convinced of the hopelessness of the woman's situation and her suffering.[38]

Case 2020-95 presented an older woman suffering from the progressive degenerative effects of Parkinson's disease. Her suffering was assessed as significant, giving warrant to MAiD and the physician's actions to provide such medical attention:

> The woman suffered from a loss of autonomy and from becoming increasingly dependent on others. She feared further experiences

of decline and regarded her situation as hopeless. Her suffering was experienced as unbearable.

The doctor, a geriatric specialist at the nursing home where the woman resided, was convinced that the suffering experienced by the woman was, by prevailing medical opinion, unbearable and without hope. [...][39]

In addition to the *Jaaverslaag 2020*, previous annual reports include similar case narratives: for example, in describing the nature of patient suffering that goads clinical euthanasia consultation, it was reported (Case 2018-68) that a 70-year-old male, with a metastatic cancer is both his lungs and brain, has been suffering from a deteriorating physical condition that threatened his autonomy, quality of life and independence. Moreover, the possibilities to remediate his suffering were determined futile. In fact, the case report put it this way: 'The patient's suffering consisted of confusion, drowsiness and urinary and faecal incontinence. He was also suffering from an increasing inability to communicate. There was nothing he was capable of doing: he could hardly walk by himself, had become bedridden and was completely dependent on others for his personal care. [...] The patient experienced his suffering as unbearable'.[40]

Another case report (Case 2017-86) identified a woman in her fifties suffering the effects of chronic obstructive pulmonary disease who had reflected on her irremediable condition:

The patient's suffering consisted of the increasing deterioration in her situation. She was experiencing severe loss of function. She could no longer eat, nor could she communicate clearly. The patient, who had always been independent, active and communicative, was entirely dependent on others and hardly able to do anything for herself. She knew there was no prospect of improvement in her situation and that the only prognosis was deterioration. She experienced her suffering as unbearable.[41]

Comparable case narratives correlate disease prognoses, futility of interventions, diminishing patient competencies and increasing dependence upon caregivers with the experiences or expressions of *uitzichtloosheid* [hopelessness].[42] For example, a man with amyotrophic lateral sclerosis, a progressive neuromuscular disease, the range of losses experienced as well as persistent pain and fear rendered his '*situatie ontluisterend* [situation humiliating]' which made of his experience unbearable.[43] For this man, it is reported (Case 2020-85) that his experience of suffering was hopeless. Suffering loss of independence and facing the spectre of being admitted to a care home, as well as fears of cognitive decline and incontinence, increasing fatigue from uncontrollable muscle tremors and other persistent symptoms of Huntington's disease, a woman in her sixties receiving palliative care (2019-123) saw her suffering as both *ondraaglijk* [unbearable] and *uitzichtloos* [hopeless].[44] For a woman in her nineties, it is recorded (Case 2018-120), 'She suffered from care dependency and the hopelessness of her situation'.[45] In Case 2018-121, it is reported that due to the disease effects and the futility of intervention, '[A man in his fifties] was bedridden and unable to do anything anymore. He has always been an active person and suffered from the shock and hopelessness of his situation. Thus, he no longer wanted to live in this way'.[46]

The persistent experience illumined by the case narratives is marked by unbearable suffering that follows the feeling that one's life is marked by '*leegte* [emptiness]' and '*het gebrek aan perspectief* [lack of perspective]' and '*reële angst* [real fear]' for some (Case 2020-102).[47] Others articulate the way persons valued '*onafhankelijkheid en zelfbeschikking* [independence and self-determination]', which become encumbered by progressions in disease and dysfunction that exaggerate losses in control over bodily agency and other declines, which are no longer wanted – even hated.[48] To '*waardig sterven* [die with dignity]'[49] is thus correlated with the kind of agency, while weakened or veiled by disease, that persons value and recite as reason for soliciting MAiD: 'Give me another universe—or I succumb. [...] Let no "feeling" disturb us ever again [...]'.[50]

Of course, it makes sense that patients might express the desire to be given a different constellation of experiences again; to recover in their lives such competencies, capacities and companions. It makes sense, meaning it is understandable, that patients confronting grievous and irremediable disease might express the dread that eventual or imminent loss of particular goods hazards. Yet so often such aims do prove unattainable and the dread is realized. Cioran paints an image of such dread so effectively, writing, 'Becoming—what a crime! Having passed through so many lungs, the air no longer renews itself. Every day vomits up its tomorrow, and I vainly try to imagine the image of a single desire. Everything is an ordeal: broken down like a beast of burden harnessed to Matter, I drag the planets'.[51]

Yet persons experiencing dread, dragging the planets, have continued to express what remains important, revealing despair. And in asking the question 'What is most important for you to achieve?' Timothy Quill and his colleagues help us to understand such despair. (Although, given Quill's reflections on and mission to secure dying with dignity, I cannot imagine that was Quill's intention[52]).

In response to this question, Quill identified four principal categories of diminishing significance, which reflected patient responses; the four categories include (1) improving quality and meaning, (2) achieving relief or comfort, (3) altering the trajectory of illness and (4) preparing for dying.[53]

Looking only at the first category, improving quality and meaning (52% of responses fit to this category), while also reiterating what we have already shown to be common to such findings, patients expressed a desire to return home, to regain function and to support significant others or not be a burden upon others.[54] Yet when unable to achieve these aims, they prove aimless; the commodities (or abstractions) of such common functional hoping, when unrealized and unachieved, prove to resource a sort of despair and the world in which these persons live becomes unbearable. Marianne Dees and her colleagues, therefore, hypothesize the following:

> While suffering is rooted in the symptoms of illness or ageing, the existential and psycho-emotional themes determine how much hope there is and whether the patient is able to bear the suffering. Unbearable suffering can only be understood in the continuum of the patient's perspectives on the past, the present, and expectations of the future. Without hopelessness, there is no perception of unbearable suffering.[55]

Conversely, where such a perception exists and persists, it does seem such persons are confronted and confounded by a particular form of hopelessness.

Let me explain further: It has been argued that life is meaningful in relation to those values or ideals that one desires to have (and fears losing). In our contemporary Western society, we value, certainly among other values, will, reason and technique. We value the exercise of individual autonomy to determine and to control the experiences and expressions of our lives. We value the concomitant technological rationality which organizes our knowing and our doing so that we might resolve particular problems and pursue practical aims – such that we might secure the artefacts essential to achieving mastery over nature and the commodities of our desires (defeating our fears). Yet such meaning-by-values leaves one vulnerable when such problems prove irresolvable, or such aims prove unreachable.

Such vulnerability risks feelings of meaninglessness. Such meaninglessness can be realized when the values for which we struggle are not there: one aims but 'aims at *nothing* and achieves *nothing*'.[56] Despair thus emerges. That is to say, despair can emerge with failed aims and unattained values.

In medicine, the diagnostic might apply as such: Autonomy and technique are such values for which both physician and patient struggle; they are characteristics of human agency we desire and think we have. Yet in the face of irremediable diagnoses, unrelenting prognoses and futile interventions where modern agencies are thwarted by the realities of frailty and finitude, the movement from a meaning-filled life to its repudiation is quick. If one cannot exercise her capacity for self-determination, or the institution of medicine cannot wield its power for controlling the mechanics of living, then our ideals have not been grasped and life made meaningful in relation to such ideals is dissolved of its value.

Despair, then, is a perspective that provokes pessimism through which the world, and its constituent parts and functions, are no longer recognised as holding value. The world 'seems worthless'.[57] While the perspective begins with seeing a possibility of realising that which we value, it concludes that we cannot. It is this conclusion, which provokes persons to despair.[58] And despair persists by both 'fear and anxiety' as Emil Cioran observes.[59] But Marcel has instructed throughout, despair grasps hold of persons caught by the unstable dialectic between desire and fear. Or, as discussed in the first chapter, 'the accumulation of (desired) possessions and the fear of losing them anew is what causes anguish and eventually despair'.[60]

Yet such despair is occluded by the promises of alleviating pain and suffering. It is occluded by the late modern narratives that insist one is free, and therefore one's authentic self, when administering will and reason as though Heracles confronting the crossroads of choice. Despair occluded by the masquerades of a hope at the crossroads, promising to deliver the 'good death' by repeating, with the assent of legal and medical opinion in a growing number of jurisdictions, the meaning-by-values that has made not only patients but also healthcare professionals and others susceptible to despair; all the while thinking it can be avoided by both reason (autonomy) and will (technique), the functions of human agency.

Fittingly, then, in the persistent chase of meaning-by-MAiD, perhaps, Cioran's reflections *on death* are apropos: 'they expect everything from the end instead of trying to grasp the meaning of a slow revelatory agony. The end will reveal too little, and they will die as ignorant as they have lived'.[61] They will die chasing meaning, which only escapes them (Ecclesiastes 2), while experiencing neither the depths nor heights of despair.[62] Instead, 'From denial to denial, his existence is diminished: [...] Liberated from what he *has* lived, unconcerned by what he *will* live, he demolishes the signposts on all his roads, and wrests himself from the dials of all time. "I shall never meet myself again", he decides [...]'.[63]

Postures of Hopelessness: Escaping Death by Death

We have previously argued the orthodoxy of autonomy and instrumental reasoning in late modernity has not only elevated the risk for persons to succumb to despair, but also serves to nourish such despair. The literature that explored the reasons for soliciting MAiD demonstrate the significance of self-determination and of control in the valuation of one's life – when persons experience threats to or the loss of these characteristics (aims or values) of autonomy and control, a persistent experience of despair emerges. Hopelessness becomes an unwelcomed existential weight as the aims that render meaning prove aimless or illusory, while tempting people towards MAiD – and back towards the orthodoxy of autonomy and instrumental reasoning. The previous two sections have therefore laboured to interrogate 'hope' for those persons confronting the limits of human finitude and the threats of frailty and death, while revealing such 'hope' as despair in disguise. The following will continue to illuminate the veiling of despair and the postures of hopelessness that persist.

Despair antagonizes human existence in that way. And it tempts relentlessly, while drawing human existence towards its annihilation: 'One [thus] cannot separate the thought of [hopeless struggle] from that of weariness and death'.[64] Put differently, those ideals most important for us risk becoming fodder for a despair, which consumes us, anticipating death. It tempts us to hug death.[65]

Such hugging of death is the posture exemplified in the modern turn towards MAiD. Such a posture is one wherein both patients and physicians, among others including family, caregivers and professionals, come to embrace death, voluntarily. Death is desired as a means to achieve another end – that is, relief from fears or problems, for example. That is, death by desire (the death of our choosing) is thought as that which offers hope. Paradoxically, this embrace of death functions as an escape from both despair and death (of that finite, fated kind). That is to say, the posture of hugging death is grounded in a pessimism nurtured, in part, by the modern desire for and fear of losing control, both individually and institutionally. MAiD affords the rational assent and clinical technique to escape the life that one does not want – the life that does not fit the arc of a Heraclean, late modern subject fighting against the problems of living and choosing against fate.

But, absurdly, choosing for death, Death can summons those desperate to escape unwanted life with 'The Rope' in hand and strewn around a neck:

> I have been waiting for you forever, I have watched your terrors, your struggles, and your rages, I have seen your rumpled sheets, the pillow where your fury gnawed, as I have heard the swearwords with which you gratified the gods. Charitable, I sympathize and offer my services. For you were born to hang yourself, like all those who disdain an answer to their doubts or an escape to their despair.[66]

That Death might be sympathetic is professed by others too – not simply by Death, itself. Consider, for example, the then Guernsey's state Deputy Rhian Tooley's conjecture concerning her mother's health was presented as justification in favour of assisted dying legislation: 'She does not cling to life, it has snagged her. It is not death which is undignified, but living after what you love in life is stripped away'.[67] That is to say, so long as despair is cultivated within the surgical theatres, doctors' offices and patient's besides of our contemporary medical milieu, suffering, loss and pain will continually render life as visibly unattractive and meaningless – as unbearable.[68] However, MAiD will be presented as the 'ace up one's sleeve' to cling to the withering strength of a desire for self-determination.[69] Thus, it seems appropriate to return to the imagery of Heracles, as late Classical accounts disclose, when he is poised to exercise heroic agency even in his death. In such accounts, he has been poisoned by deceit[70] and left alone to build a funeral pyre, to drag *himself* to its pinnacle, only to command final aid to relieve his suffering by setting the pyre ablaze.[71]

We can see that patients are vulnerable to such despair, as proposed above. Yet they are conditioned also by desires for self-determination and technological rationalities that are retold by professionals, policies and legislation. The withering patient, inundated by despair, imagines the clinical administration of death as the only remaining act of control.[72] It determines a response: Death is the right thing *to do*.

So now, in many jurisdictions, for the individual hugging her own death, being hugged *by* Death, medical services are offered to aid her despair, affirming her judgement while also reinforcing illusions of self-control. This is done whilst safeguarding the illusion of meaning and control for the physician and the physicians guild, because of the capacity to bring forth death by will. Or, as Philoctetes willed to set the funeral pyre ablaze, relieving Heracles of his torment, the physician and the physician's guild emerge, stand readied to slay the anxieties and intolerabilities of life in the midst of death. Another hero, thus, ascends ready to hug the death of the other – all the while arguing he does so according to his traditional commitment to the patient, thus on behalf of and in service to the triumph of autonomy.

While the imagery of standing at the ready might conjure heroic imagery, all might not be as heroic. There are those, after all, who might also wield *Death as a power*,[73] not only affirming the judgement of those in the depths of despair, but also condemning others whose state is incompatible with contemporary ideals conformed by technological rationalities and expressions of autonomy. Consider, for example, the inflammatory words of the late British philosopher Baroness Mary Warnock, as reported in *The Times*, regarding those persons suffering dementia: 'you're wasting people's lives – your family's lives – and you're wasting the resources of the National Health Service'.[74] Warnock went on to argue, such persons have a 'duty to die'.[75]

And an unnamed physician now in possession of the poisoned arrows of Heracles was culpable to ensure such a duty (described as a previous self-expression of desire) was fulfilled in the Netherlands, as one might have read in both *The Guardian* and *The Telegraph*.[76] (Of course, the arrows were now a sedative 'slipped' into the patient's coffee followed by further rounds of sedatives that proved ineffective and the administration of lethal medicine, which was not injected until family successfully restrained the patient).[77] Acquitted of charges, the defence relied heavily upon the apparatus of (respect for) autonomy at work in biomedical ethics: As conveyed by Christopher de Bellaigue in *The Guardian*, 'she was fulfilling her patient's request and that, since the patient was incompetent, her protests before her death were irrelevant'.[78] The judges agreed, the medic acted in the correct manner – fulfilled her functions and 'freed [the patient] from the mental prison which she ended up in'.[79] And Steven Pleiter, the former director of the *Expertisecentrum Euthanasie*, implicitly supports the actions of the unnamed physician, hoping 'the most complex varieties of euthanasia, like psychiatric illnesses and dementia' will be found acceptable.[80] After all, drawing upon a technological imperative, Pleiter continued: 'If the situation is unbearable and there is no prospect of improvement, and euthanasia is an option, it would be almost unethical [of a doctor] not to *help* that person'.[81]

Some might suggest that such help is heroic and the cheers in the Dutch courts upon hearing of the acquittal evidence the *good* of such actions. Perhaps not. Perhaps the present milieu of MAiD is, as discussed, cultivated from despair and the cheers simply smother reality. And if so, it is woefully dreadful. After all, if suffering, loss and pain encumbers the modern subject *and* thus renders life as unsightly and morose, as having no worth, such rejection of existence, inescapable to despair, is not only a valuation of the self (or another) as being worth less, but also a judgment that I am (or Thou is) worth less for others. It is akin to stating that life is wholly disposable and utterly unworthy of existence in a particular present state because of its functional, often rational, encumbrances or impediments.

Thus, the potent allure of the modern subject and the corresponding promises of technological rationalities incumbent to our late modern milieu does seem to hazard derision and a determinative logic wrought from despair. The logic might be as such: Bereft of choices, bereft of a particular understanding of being and of freedom, we would, it is argued, prefer to exercise by medical means a final will to self-determine, our 'right' or our duty to die. Others, therefore, argue that we have been so formed by the late modern project that persons often cannot get out from under the imperative for autonomy and the corresponding technological rationality. Some go so far to suggest that such persons are paradoxically enslaved by its appeal. Carol Stoneking is one such person, offering the provocative assessment:

> Our society is so captive to the notion of control that we imagine we ought to control our own deaths; thus physician-assisted suicide is nothing if not cooperation born of the desire to secure the 'best outcome'. Belief in human autonomy, rather than belief in God, is the background belief that makes a positive description of suicide or euthanasia possible. Autonomy has become an imperative; that which we cannot control, our belief in autonomy teaches us to hate. Thus, we learn to hate our aging bodies; and we learn to hate those others who are sick and dying. We even learn to hate those we would define as 'permanently dependent', exactly because they will always need our care.[82]

So, although the conjecture of a moral philosopher and actions of a Dutch physician might seem an outlier and Stoneking's logic of 'hate' might sound hyperbolic, the bioethics literature does point towards increasing support for MAiD. Moreover, it does point towards an increasing endorsement of MAiD not only for those persons who command their death, as Heracles commands Philoctetes, but also for persons suffering various grades of dementia and unable to utter such a command due to restrictions of competence and capacity. And some, like Steven Pleiter, *hope* that 'acceptance [...] grows and grows over the years'.[83]

In 1998, for example, an American study surveyed the public ($N = 447$, aged ≥ 65 years) and revealed that approximately 11% accepted medically assisted dying for persons with mild dementia.[84] A 1999 Australian survey of registered nurses ($N = 1220$), 39% supported the legislation of euthanasia for patients with mild dementia.[85] While two different studies from the Netherlands in 1998 and 2013 revealed significant support for medical assistance in dying for persons suffering dementia. Joop van Hosteyn and Margo Trappenburg surveyed the public ($N = 911$), revealing 48% supported euthanasia for severe dementia, if requested whilst a person was capable.[86] While Pauline Kouwenhoven and her colleagues, using mixed methodologies, showed variable opinions depending on grade of dementia: Among the general public ($N = 1960$), 24% supported physician assistance and 77% supported euthanasia for persons with mild and advanced dementia, respectively; among health professionals ($N = 1243$, nurses; $N = 793$, physicians), 28% of physicians and 31% of nurses supported physician assistance in dying while 33% of physicians and 58% of nurses supported euthanasia for those with mild and advanced dementia, respectively.[87] Finally, a 2006 study in the Netherland revealed that 74% of carers ($N = 36$) agreed that euthanasia is permissible for patients suffering late-stage dementia when accompanied by advanced directive while a 2007 study in the United Kingdom revealed approximately 44% to nearly 60% of persons surveyed from the general public ($N = 725$) would support medical assistance in dying for themselves or their partners with mild to severe dementia.[88]

Acceptance of such action is one thing. That the *Second Annual Report on MAiD in Canada 2020*, for example, gives an accounting of 30 individuals with Alzheimer's disease or dementia (approximately 4% of cases reported) who participated in MAiD is yet another. That the report does not clarify how it was that these persons were 'always able to provide' for the moral and legal standard of informed consent remains a question for those surveying the eligibility and safeguard standards of MAiD in Canada.[89] The Canadian Broadcasting Company's (CBC) The Sunday Edition radio documentary, 'Ten-Minutes to Midnight', however, might provide some indication of how and where the safeguards might be catalysed to lower the threshold for participation in MAiD.[90]

Perhaps the metaphor of a catalyst here is unnecessary, since another metaphor is introduced in this documentary, which might be sufficiently explanatory. Using a developmental metaphor, Stefanie Green, the head of the Canadian Association of MAiD Assessors and Providers (CAMAP), discusses the interpretation of the law and MAiD services concerning eligibility and safeguards as a process of *maturation*.[91] So, when persons with dementia meet the criteria that delimits the law and limits abuses, Green believes such persons should be deemed eligible. And for Green, her opinion here is not positioned as unique, but argued to be indicative of the 'majority of providers in this country', who too have concluded that 'patients with dementia can be assessed for an assisted death, that some of them may be eligible in certain circumstances, and if that is the case, they'd be willing to help them'.[92]

Green's decision to provide MAiD services to Gayle Garlock, one of the first Canadians to acquire such services while suffering dementia and its deleterious effects. Green's testimony in the CBC radio documentary pressed into the question of competence, which remains a limit to accessing MAiD services in Canada. At present, persons cannot carry through with MAiD services if assessed as incompetent, even when the request was made previously while competent. Thus, Green's emphasis that she had determined Gayle to be competent, again and again, and to be suffering unbearably was of critical legal import. But her emphasis came with a qualification regarding competence, which functions as a kind of apology for a revision to (or a recognized maturing of) Canadian legislation as well as a call for medical providers to consider competence provisionally, and often, during the extended event associated with the protracted MAiD protocol between service request and provision.

A revision of legislation accepted, what then does one make of such data, opinion and anecdote in light of the argument thus far? One might turn again to the ways the modern subject and the ideals of our technological society have coerced a particular disposition incumbent to the broken work – familiar to the problematic life. But such repetition is not necessary here.

Perhaps it is better to think of physicians and nurses and carers as we might consider Deianira: Deceived by a story of potions and powers, she had a blood-smeared cloak placed upon her husband Heracles. While intending to secure fidelity, Deianira unwittingly adorned him with anguish and hastened his death. Of course, this might simply stretch the comparison too far.

Death as Clinical Problem, Dying as a Human Experience

No matter what one makes of the argument thus far, people increasingly agree that 'Death is a clinical phenomenon', which medical professionals know well.[93] That is to suggest, the institution of medicine and its corresponding understanding of the human body has judiciously attended to the mechanisms of human life, including those that correspond with death and dying. I wouldn't disagree, necessarily. Yet, Marcel might suggest the repeated observations of such mechanisms has educated medical practitioners to observe persons as mere objects. I wouldn't disagree necessarily with this suggestion, either. Jeffrey Bishop, after all, has argued convincingly of something similar. Such a disposition risks producing practitioners, as Bishop laments, who are 'forgetful of meaning and purpose'[94] – which reflects Gillian Rose's accusation in the introduction. Marcel simply admits, the perspective of such practitioners disciplined by the habits of the 'technical world, with its compass set in a direction, can only end in despair'.[95] As we have seen above, it is certainly possible that the lives of those persons suffering the devastations of irremediable disease are vulnerable to end in despair too; but holding onto death as a readied answer – certain of the resolution to a problematic life.

To be sure, the institution of medicine does concern itself with a particular understanding of meaning and purpose. Yet, the response to the questions raised within the milieu of medicine concerned with the *problems* of life (and of death) is not one in which meaning and purpose is explored most fully. What medical professionals understand well are the various modalities and mechanics that one might introduce to regulate human physiology about homeostatic means as well as the skills and practical interventions shown reliable to assuage harmful pathologies. That is to suggest that medical professionals understand very well how to poke and to prod the human body, exciting its parts to function as though a mechanic reviving an automobile. And patients trust these *bio*-mechanics to ensure that their functions for self-making and independent actions can persist.

'But', as Donald MacKinnon has enquired further, 'is [death] only that?'[96] Is death merely a problem to be resolved by the meaning-making practices of a technocratic health system and the persons (both patients and professionals) wielding constituent parts to maintain the functions for the continued motion of matter? MacKinnon probes even further, raising similar questions as Bishop: '[H]ave we anything to learn from poetry, from the language of religion, and so on? [...] Is it or is it not true that those who still mouth the logical vulgarities of traditional arguments concerning immortality do so because in the end they just cannot allow that the clinician has said or can say all that is to be significantly said about death?'[97]

The short answer is, 'No!' Life and death, ageing and dying, are not simply *problems* that can be managed to suit desires through technological means. We cannot separate ourselves from the embodied lives we live. The human condition includes existential dimensions beyond the grasp of pure technique or primary reflection (as Marcel repeats).

While humanists might not have the knowledge over the clinical phenomenon of death, they confront it intellectually as an existential question, which is often an integral part of the dying process in the clinical context but for which clinicians are not necessarily equipped often to address. Furthermore, humanists contribute to and foster reflections about the art of living well in the face of mortality and human finitude.[98] The field of medical humanities precisely invites such scholarly endeavours but as this book has demonstrated thus far, the narratives of late modernity and the *sclerotic unavailability*[99] it conditions discourages or challenges, if not undermines, the inclusion of these important insights – insights that have no evident use.

MacKinnon's question on the limits of clinical knowing pleads for us to explore further the disposition incumbent to modern medicine, which labours to uncover the meaning-making practice of *doing* against death, a problem to be resolved. Through such exploration, however, the preceding has highlighted the particular anxieties, fears and preoccupations of the broken world, while attempting to demonstrate the subsequent disposition towards ageing and dying as necessarily limiting and, ultimately, destructive.

Human life and death, ageing and dying, pain and suffering, are mere epistemological problems to be conquered by medical conquest purchased by power gained by the objectifying distance from that over which such knowing is to be exerted. And there is a habituated certainty in such knowing. That is, there is stereotyped response. It is a response to the anguish experienced, desiring a 'good death', fearing a terrible fate. There is stereotyped response to 'dream of escape' and 'run'.

It is a stereotyped response which permits control but risks experiencing the fulness of the human condition. It is a stereotyped response that promises to deliver a hope, but such hope is merely a repetition of aims that offer up despair but in disguise.

There must be another way to live, grow old and die. There must be another way, because 'I am going to die' too. We all are.

There is. But *the way* is a mystery for wayfarers.

Notes

1 While I've introduced this person previously, Patricia's impact on the trajectory of my academic interests and vocation have proven significant. It's right to remember her here again. See Ashley John Moyse, *Reading Karl Barth, Interrupting Moral Technique, Transforming Biomedical Ethics* (New York: Palgrave, 2015), 1–2.

2 I'm using 'mystery' as informed by Gabriel Marcel and as introduced within the introduction. As a reminder, for Marcel, 'the *mystery of being* involves the active situation that we are concerned with—our experiences—and so, is one whose true nature can only be grasped, acknowledged, or recognized from the inside' (Hernandez, *Marcel's Ethics of Hope*, 13). And in her situation, the recognition that she experiences the healthy and sick life of her body (and soul), as introduced in the first chapter, without abstraction, refusing to offer an accounting that tabulates gains or losses of the things of life one has/had as on a ledger, offers a lived example of Marcel's understanding/experience of mystery. That she turned towards others inviting the sharing of joy, will be shown as the groundwork of being and of hope in the final chapter. That she, even in her state, proved responsible for me was a humanising revelation.

3 A. A. Gill, *Sunday Times*, 20 November (2016); As quoted by O'Mahony, *Can Medicine Be Cured*, 149.

4 O'Mahony, *Can Medicine Be Cured*, 151. Writing about 'hope' for the treatment of Cancer, O'Mahony recalls the 'childlike enthusiasm' Christopher Hitchens expressed for similar immunotherapies and other experimental stem cell treatment interventions. Similarly, O'Mahony discusses the case of Susan Sontag, who also had expressed trust in the science of modern oncology and the oncologists, themselves. For O'Mahony, such trust is misguided, for what he can see from within the halls of hospital and hospice, 'Cancer treatment (in addition to being unaffordable and unsustainable in many circumstances) seems to offer some patients a toxic combination of false hopes and a bad death' (Seamus O'Mahony, 'Celebrity Cancer Ward', in *The Way We Die Now* (London: Head of Zeus, 2017), 142–179 (170).

5 Critchley, *Notes on Suicide*, 63.

6 Marc Etkind, ed., *...Or Not to Be: A Collection of Suicide Notes* (New York: Riverhead, 1997), 101.

7 'About Us', Death with Dignity, https://deathwithdignity.org/about/. Accessed 21 July 2021.

8 Etkind, *Or Not to Be*, 107.

9 Russell Aldwinckle, *Death in the Secular City* (London: George Allen & Unwin, 1972).

10 As the experience is retold, Jack Kevorkian said 'Have a nice trip' to Janet Adkins as she turned on his 'Thanatron', the death machine used to produce death for his 'patients' (Etkind, *Or Not to Be*, 100).

11 Emil Cioran writes of 'Annihilation by Deliverance', saying: 'Salvation ends everything; and ends us. Who, once *saved*, dares still call himself alive?' (Cioran, *Short History of Decay*, 29). It ends everything for at least the one—the one who 'shall never meet [oneself] again' (64). Yet 'incarceration, humiliation, disappointment, disease' remain realities for others; suffering rages on (Critchley, *Notes on Suicide*, 72).

12 Critchley, *Notes on Suicide*, 73.

13 Tom Beauchamp, 'The Right to Die as the Triumph of Autonomy', *Journal of Medicine and Philosophy* 31 (2006): 643–654 (644, 651).

14 Mortimer, 'The Triumph of the Doctors', 97–116.

15 As reported by Christopher de Bellaigue, 'Death on demand: Has euthanasia gone too far?', *The Guardian* (18 January 2019). Retrieved at https://www.theguardian.com/news/2019/jan/18/death-on-demand-has-euthanasia-gone-too-far-netherlands-assisted-dying?CMP=ShareiOSAppOther&fbclid=IwAR3FHnMkBs-cboxgzVOLZ81a8hhYMCEc77e6wT4JuJN8sQyRdwugUFRe3K4. Expertisecentrum Euthanasie (Expertise Centre Euthanasia, https://expertisecentrumeuthanasie.nl) was formerly called *Levenseindekliniek* (End of Life Clinic), as reported by de Ballaigue, before a name change in 2019.

16 Kurt Goldstein, 'Health as value', in *New Knowledge in Human Values*, ed. Abraham Maslow (New York: Harper, 1959), 178–188; John Bruhn and George Henderson, *Values in Health Care: Choices and Conflict* (Springfield: Charles C. Thomas, 1991).

17 Michael Banner, 'Scripts for Modern Dying: The Death before Death We Have Invented, the Death before Death We Fear and Some Take Too Literally, and the Death before Death Christians Believe In', *Studies in Christian Ethics* 29, no. 3 (2016): 249–255.

18 Daniel Callahan, Daniel, 'The WHO definition of health', *The Hastings Center Studies* 1, no. 3 (1973): 77–88 (82–83).

19 Christopher Braider, 'Hercules at the Crossroads: Image and soliloquy in Annibale Carracci', In *Iconoclasm: Turning Toward Pictures*, ed. Ellen Spolsky 89–116 (Lewisburg: Bucknell University Press, 2014), 89–116 (89).

20 Vivian Sleight, 'Hope and Despair', *Journal of the Royal Society of Medicine* 97 (2004): 354.

21 Ibid., 354.

22 Ibid., 354

23 Ovid. *Metamorphoses*, Anthony S Kline (Trans.), Bk IX.159-210. Retrieved from http://ovid.lib.virginia.edu/trans/Ovhome.htm

24 Commission fédérale de Contrôle et d'Évaluation de l'Euthanasie, 'Communiqué de presse: EUTHANASIE—Chiffres de l'année 2020' [Commission for the Control and Evaluation of Euthanasia, 'Press Release: "EUTHANASIA—Figures for the Year 2020']. Retrieved at https://organesdeconcertation.sante.belgique.be/sites/default/files/documents/cfcee_chiffres-2020_communiquepresse.pdf

25 Commission Nationale de Contrôle et d'Évaluation de l'application de la loi du 16 mars 2009 sur l'euthanasie et l'assistance au suicide, 'Cinquième rapport à l'attention de la Chambre des Députés (années 2017 et 2018)' [National Commission for the Control and Evaluation of the Application of the Law of 16 March 2009 on Euthanasia and Assisted Suicide, Fifth report for the attention of the Chamber of Deputies (years 2017 and 2018)]: 13. Retrieved at https://sante.public.lu/fr/publications/r/rapport-loi-euthanasie-2017-2018/rapport-loi-euthanasie-2017-2018.pdf

26 'Table 1. Characteristics and end-of-life care of 1,905 DWDA patients who have died from ingesting a lethal dose of medication as of 22 January 2021, Oregon, 1998–2020', Oregon Death With Dignity Act Data Summary, (February 2021): 12. Retrieved at https://www.oregon.gov/oha/PH/PROVIDERPARTNERRESOURCES/EVALUATIONRESEARCH/DEATHWITHDIGNITYACT/Documents/year23.pdf.

27 'Table 2. End of life concerns of participants who died, 2016–2018', Washington State 2018 Death with Dignity Act Report, (July 2019): 11. Retrieved at https://www.doh.wa.gov/Portals/1/Documents/Pubs/422-109-DeathWithDignityAct2018.pdf.

28 '4.3 Nature of Suffering of Those Who Received MAID', *Second Annual Report on Medical Assistance in Dying in Canada, 2020* (Ottawa: Health Canada, 2021), 19–20. Retrieved at https://www.canada.ca/content/dam/hc-sc/documents/services/medical-assistance-dying/annual-report-2020/annual-report-2020-eng.pdf

29 Linda Ganzini, Elizabeth R. Goy and Stephen K. Dobscha, 'Why Oregon Patients Request Assisted Death: Family Members' Views', *Journal of General Internal Medicine* 23, no. 2 (2008): 154–157; Bryant Carlson, et al., 'Oregon Hospice Chaplains' Experiences with Patients Requesting Physician-Assisted Suicide', *Journal of Palliative Medicine* 8, no. 6 (2005): 1160–1166; Linda Ganzini, et al., 'Oregon Physicians' Perceptions of Patients Who Request Assisted Suicide and Their Families', *Journal of Palliative Medicine* 6, no. 3 (2003): 381–390; Linda Ganzini, et al., 'Experiences of Oregon Nurses and Social Workers with Hospice Patients Who Requested Assistance with Suicide', *New England Journal of Medicine* 347, no. 8 (2002): 582–588; Linda Ganzini, et al., 'Physicians' Experiences with the Oregon Death with Dignity Act', *New England Journal of Medicine* 342, no. 8 (2000): 557–563.

30 Linda Ganzini, Elizabeth R. Goy and Stephen K. Dobscha, 'Oregonians' Reasons for Requesting Physician Aid in Dying', *Archives of Internal Medicine* 169, no. 5 (2009): 489–493.

31 Robert A. Pearlman, et al., 'Motivations for Physician-assisted Suicide: Patient and Family Voices', *Journal of Gerontology and Internal Medicine*, vol. 20 (2005): 234–239.

32 Maggie Hendry, et al., 'Why Do We Want the Right to Die? A Systematic Review of the International Literature on the Views of Patients, Carers, and the Public on Assisted Dying', *Palliative Medicine* 27, no. 1 (2012): 13–26.

33 Marianne K. Dees, et al., '"Unbearable Suffering": A Qualitative Study on the Perspectives of Patients Who Request Assistance in Dying', *Journal of Medical Ethics* 37, no. 12 (2011): 727–734 (732).

34 Ibid., 732.

35 Ibid., 732.

36 These statements have been collated from Martina Pestinger, et al., 'The Desire to Hasten Death: Using Grounded Theory for a Better Understanding 'When Perception of Time Tends to be a Slippery Slope'', *Palliative Medicine* 29, no. 8 (2015): 711–719 (714).

37 You can retrieve all reports (some with English translations), dating from 2002, through the following URL provided: https://www.euthanasiecommissie.nl/de-toetsingscommissies/jaarverslagen.

38 Regionale Toetsingscommissies Euthanasie, 'Jaarverslag 2020', (April 2020): 32. Translation is mine.

39 Ibid., 34. Translation is mine.

40 Regionale Toetsingscommissies Euthanasie, 'Jaarverslag 2018', (April 2019): 28–29 (Translated provided, 'Annual Report 2018', 26–27).

41 Regionale Toetsingscommissies Euthanasie, 'Jaarverslag 2017', (April 2018): 32 (Translation provided, 'Annual Report 2018', 29).

42 Interestingly, while the original Dutch works use *uitzichtloosheid* in their case reports, for example, the English translations do not. A cumbersome euphemism, noting there to be no prospect of improvement, is used in the translations.

43 'Jaarverslag 2020', 39. Translation is mine.

44 Regionale Toetsingscommissies Euthanasie, 'Jaarverslag 2019', (April 2020): 35. Translation is mine. As noted above, 'hopelessness' is not included in the English report. Instead, the translation indicates that the woman suffered 'the lack of any prospect of improvement' (Translation provided, 'Annual Report 2019', 35).

45 'Jaarverslag 2018', 43. Translation is mine.

46 Ibid., 46.

47 'Jaarverlag 2020', 36. Translation is mine.

48 Ibid., 37.

49 Ibid., 37.

50 Cioran, *Short History of Decay*, 126.

51 Ibid., 126.

52 See Timothy E. Quill, 'Death and Dignity', *New England Journal of Medicine* 324, no. 10 (1991): 691–694; Jane Gross, 'Quiet Doctor Finds a Mission in Assisted Suicide Court Case', *New York Times*, (2 January 1997): B1. Retrieved August 2021, https://www.nytimes.com/1997/01/02/nyregion/quiet-doctor-finds-a-mission-in-assisted-suicide-court-case.html

53 Timothy Quill, et al., 'What Is Most Important for You to Achieve? An Analysis of Patient Responses When Receiving Palliative Care Consultation', *Journal of Palliative Medicine* 9, no. 2 (2006): 382–388.

54 Ibid., 384.

55 Dees, 'Unbearable Suffering', 733.

56 Nietzsche, *Will to Power*, 12.

57 Ibid., 22.

58 Nietzsche, *Thus Spoke Zarathustra*, 228.

59 Cioran, *Heights of Despair*, 19.

60 O'Callaghan, 'Hope and Freedom', 218.

61 Cioran, *Heights of Despair*, 27.

62 Ibid., 37–38.

63 Cioran, *Short History of Decay*, 64.

64 Cioran, *Heights of Despair*, 16.

65 Marcel, *Being and Having*, 37–38.

66 Cioran, *Short History of Decay*, 157.

67 Steven Morris, '"Right thing to do": Guernsey begins assisted dying debate', *The Guardian*, 16 May 2018, para 20. Retrieved from https://www.theguardian.com/society/2018/may/16/right-thing-to-do-guernsey-begins-assisted-dying-debate

68 Dees, et al., 'Unbearable suffering', 727–734

69 Cristina Monforte-Royo, et al., 'What Lies Behind the Wish to Hasten Death? A Systematic Review and Meta-Ethnography from the Perspective of Patients', *PLoS ONE*, vol. 7, no. 5 (2012): e371117 (1–16).

70 Poisoned by the blood of the deceptive centaur Nessus. Nessus was killed by Heracles' poisoned arrows after assaulting his wife, Deianira. Nessus, while dying gave Deianira his blood saying it was a potent love potion. So, when Heracles brought

home as a concubine the beautiful Iole, the young daughter of his archery master, whom he killed in revenge for not giving of his daughter earlier, Deianira thought of the blood as a guarantee. By its application, Heracles' love for her would remain steadfast. Thus, the blood was smeared upon a cloak, which Deianira placed upon Heracles' shoulders. Unable to remove the cloak, the poisonous blood, like an acid through metal, consumed his flesh (Ovid, Bk IX, 89–158, 159–210).

71 Ovid, BK IX 159–210, 211–272.

72 See Monforte-Royo, et al., 'What Lies Behind the Wish to Hasten Death?'

73 William Stringfellow, 'The Moral Reality Named Death', in *An Ethic for Christians and Other Aliens in a Strange Land* (Eugene: Wipf & Stock, 2004), 67–94.

74 As quoted by Martin Beckford, 'Baroness Warnock: Dementia sufferers may have a duty to die', *The Telegraph*, 18 September 2008. Retrieved from http://www.telegraph.co.uk/news/uknews/2983652/Baroness-Warnock-Dementia-sufferers-may-have-a-duty-to-die.html

75 Ibid.

76 Daniel Boffey, 'Doctor to face prosecution for breach of euthanasia law', *The Guardian*, 9 November 2018. Retrieved from https://www.theguardian.com/world/2018/nov/09/doctor-to-face-dutch-prosecution-for-breach-of-euthanasia-law; Senay Boztas, 'Dutch doctor reprimanded for 'asking family to hold down euthanasia patient'', *The Telegraph*, 25 July 2018. Retrieved from https://www.telegraph.co.uk/ news/2018/07/25/dutch-doctor-reprimanded-asking-family-hold-euthanasia-patient/

77 Daniel Boffey, 'Dutch doctor acquitted in landmark euthanasia case', *The Guardian*, 11 September 2019. Retrieved from https://www.theguardian.com/world/2019/sep/11/dutch-court-clears-doctor-in-landmark-euthanasia-trial

78 de Bellaigue, 'Death on demand'.

79 A phrase the daughter uttered while referring to her mother and in support of the physician, as quoted by Boffey, 'Dutch doctor acquitted'.

80 As quoted by de Belaigue, 'Death on demand'.

81 Ibid. Emphasis is mine.

82 Carole Bailey Stoneking, 'Receiving Communion: Euthanasia, Suicide, and Letting Die', in *The Blackwell Companion to Christian Ethics*, edited by Stanley Hauerwas and Samuel Wells, 375–387 (Malden: Blackwell, 2006), 382.

83 As quoted by de Bellaigue, 'Death on demand', 36.

84 Victor G. Cicirelli, 'Views of elderly people concerning end-of-life decisions', *Journal of Applied Gerontology* 17, no. 2 (1998): 186–203.

85 Betty Kitchener and Anthony F. Jorm, 'Conditions required for a law on active voluntary euthanasia: a survey of nurses' opinions in the Australian Capital Territory', *Journal of Medical Ethics* 25, no. 1 (1999): 25–30.

86 Joop van Holsteyn and Margo Trappenburg, 'Citizens' opinions on new forms of euthanasia: A report from the Netherlands', *Patient Education and Counseling* 35, no. 1 (1998): 63–73.

87 Pauline S. C. Kouwenhoven, et al., 'Opinions of health care professionals and the public after eight years of euthanasia legislation in the Netherlands: A mixed methods approach', *Palliative Medicine* 27, no. 9 (2013): 273–280.

88 Mette L. Rurup, et al., 'Attitudes of physicians, nurses and relatives towards end-of-life decisions concerning nursing home patients with dementia', *Patient Education and Counseling* 61, no. 3 (2006): 372–380; Nia Williams, et al., 'Public attitudes to

life- sustaining treatments and euthanasia in dementia', *International Journal of Geriatric Psychiatry* 22, no. 12 (2007): 1229–1234.

89 *Second Annual Report on Medical Assistance in Dying in Canada, 2020* (Ottawa: Health Canada, 2021), 17.

90 'Ten-Minutes to Midnight', by Alisa Siegel (Prod.) and Karen Levine (Ed.), The Sunday Edition, *CBC Radio* (32.27min), 27 October 2019, https://www.cbc.ca/radio/sunday/the-sunday-edition-for-october-27-2019-1.5335017/b-c-man-is-one-of-the-first-canadians-with-dementia-to-die-with-medical-assistance-1.5335025. Accessed 10 July 2021.

91 Ibid., 26:10–26:38.

92 Ibid., 26:18–26:37.

93 Donald MacKinnon, 'Death (1955)', in *Philosophy and the Burden of Theological Honesty: A Donald MacKinnon Reader*, ed. John C McDowell (London: T&T Clark, 2011), 307–311 (308).

94 Bishop, *Anticipatory Corpse*, 119.

95 Marcel, *Man Against Mass Society*, 71.

96 MacKinnon, 'Death', 308.

97 Ibid., 309.

98 I can't think of any better a recent book than that of Lydia Dugdale, whose *The Lost Art of Dying* works to do just this very thing. As Dugdale commends, 'If the art of dying well is in truth the art of living well, then how ought we to live? How might we face death and still flourish? The ancient Greek philosophers Plato and Aristotle thought that if you wanted to do anything well, you had – at the very least – to live a life of virtue. [...] The tendency to despair as death approaches can be remedied through a lifetime of exercise hopefulness' (Lydia S. Dugdale, *The Lost Art of Dying: Reviving Forgotten Wisdom* (New York: HarperOne, 2020), 203–204). Of course, as we will see in the following chapter, Dugdale might find good company alongside Marcel – but he might challenge 'remedy' and suggest 'triumph', which does not necessarily remove the actuality of despair as a persistent passion through which the wayfarer journey hopefully.

99 Marcel, 'Ontological Mystery', 40–41.

Chapter 4

WAYFARING THROUGH DESPAIR, PRACTISING HOPE

From the outset, that task has been to study a particular imaginary (among others that have given shape to the modern project as well as the individual and social preoccupations to transform the world to one that is controllable). Thinking with Marcel, this particular imaginary is one where persons become problems for themselves – where persons come to think that 'existence is a problem to be solved' through the administration and continued exercise of vital and social functions which can be deployed in order to possess our desires and to assuage our fears.[1] Running from the actualities of corporeality and experiences of suffering (coming to regard them 'from the outside' as purely objective phenomena, or problems, to be studied, subdued and surmounted by way of technique), we discovered persons perceiving a broken world. 'From the outside', frail ageing and terminal diagnoses are regarded as objectively delimited impediments to achieving particular and, often, technologically mediated, aims or ideals (like the freedom from pain and suffering). However, we have also seen, frailty and illness, including depredations of ageing and dying, do prove relentless and the problematical reveals itself as fodder for despair. Additionally, pessimism has been revealed by a constellation of functional hopes; a pessimism that admits life *is* meaningless when late modern ideals, including control, independence, autonomy and the like, are threatened, unobtained or lost. We have, therefore, encountered a perspective that seeks after relief from such despair, but remains unable to see another way beyond the world of the problematical.

Unwittingly perhaps, persons, both young and old, do believe that overcoming death is a principal and possible and good goal of medicine. Ageing, considered as a pathology that leads to death, like a cancer or virus or bacterium, is thus a *thing* like any other, which we can eradicate from human experience with the right kind of technique. Dying too can be domesticated by managed options elected by the living, which serve to overcome the fated ugliness of death (that death which offends our agency and desire). Perhaps these same persons do prioritise living over dying. Perhaps they do so happily, faith-filled that pain and suffering and the disorder of ageing and dying *are* discrete states that ought to, and therefore can, be eliminated. They think:

> The only thing that exists are states, which are either desirable or undesirable. Those that are not desirable, i.e., the states of suffering, are to be eliminated, and if there is no other way, then this rejection is to be achieved by eliminating the one who suffers. For the sufferer does not in reality have an actuality, a being, that would be something more than the sum of the conditions in which it happens to be. It is not in fact someone who suffers, but it is suffering that demands to be eliminated from reality.[2]

And so, the logic that has cultivated despair turns to a repetition, which futilely clamours for meaning – by the strength of desire (fear) and technique, confronting the persistence of pain and suffering, we must eliminate that which we do not want to have from reality, anticipating particular managed, programmatic efforts to overcome such depredations – including suicide by one's own hand or by the hand of another (death as a means to overcome an unwanted reality).

Such actions labour to kill that *thing*, or those several things, we have come to hate – the hated objects forced upon the functionalised lives we have, whether depredations, diseases, or dependencies. And when programmatic efforts prove futile and options to choose prove few, we encounter a familiar *apologia*, which can become as repetitions of this man's suicide note: 'I'm done with life/I'm no good/I'm dead'.[3] Or, as introduced in the Chapter 2, the dissatisfaction with life (or future life) delimits a readiness to 'give up': Collecting interviews from 25 people in later life (an average age of 85 years) but without terminal or mental illness who believed their lives to be 'completed' or no longer worth living, Els van Wijngaarden's research reveals a range of 'curses'[4] that exaggerate the existential anxieties of living, rendering a perspective through which persons become dissatisfied with and readied to end life. These include loneliness, feeling insignificant and ineffective in communication, inundated by both existential and physical fatigue, and averse to feared dependence.[5] (Of course, all of these can and often are experienced by persons throughout the whole of life; that our broken world makes of these experiences mere problems to overcome while narratives of self-sufficiency predominate, it seems we are tormented at every age by a vulnerability to despair). These states are thought to be as those which ought to be eliminated but remain, stimulating thinking that life is no longer worth living as it is currently experienced.

A note from a woman who was suffering from multiple sclerosis might be indicative of the kind of state that is thought to claim action in order to secure relief (to secure that 'hope' for relief, which Vivien Sleight introduced in the Chapter 3):

'I'm bored with my bodily functions and my mind is going. It's better to end it now while I can still do something'.[6] The body, in this instance, is objectively functionalised – these functions of the body, along with particular functions of mind, are the problems upon which this woman's gaze had been fixated. And *having* the body in this way, in a broken world, means that one has come to think she has a power over it – no matter how illusory such control might be.[7]

But pain and suffering are not illusions. Yet our late modern or broken world, filled with its problems, is preoccupied with narratives that discipline imaginations to civilize the world of our desires and to train us to say that we can, by incumbent rationalities and concomitant techniques, control objective, functionalised experiences and expressions, or, as Spaemann has delimited above, states of pain and suffering. We thus learn to see pain and suffering as meaningful when they are absent – and we learn to see ourselves as possessing meaning when we achieve control over such pain and suffering. Yet when uncontrolled, or when hope for control is thwarted, fear, anguish and despair emerge as the world of our aims proves aimless; and the panoptic gaze of such nihilism risks turning inward, where persons come to judge themselves also as worthless too.[8] This kind of *meaning* must be resisted.

Thankfully, we have exemplars of resistance. The writings of Ivan Illich and his own experiences with illness are representative of such resistance.[9] His resistance, enabled by a lifetime of preparation,[10] is bolstered by a cantankerous spirit raised against the (late) modern medical milieu that has been disciplined by technique. Illich is profoundly critical when suffering loses its dignity as it becomes disciplined by the pursuits of health delimited maximally as 'complete physical, mental and social wellbeing' – or the pursuits of 'a system not yet perfect but decisively aimed at perfection'.[11] Homogenized by the technocratic imaginary, which Marcel might discuss as degradation of mass, technocratic society,[12] 'Medical civilization is planned and organized to kill pain, to eliminate sickness, and to abolish the need for *an art of suffering and of dying*.'[13] Illich continues, writing, 'This progressive flattening out of personal, virtuous performance constitutes a new goal which has never before been a guideline for social life. Suffering, healing, and dying [...] are now claimed by technocracy as new areas of policy-making and are treated as malfunctions from which populations ought to be institutionally relieved.'[14]

Such planning and organisation, such flattening out by biomedicine and the incumbent rationalities of the broken world, Illich 'demonstrated the art of suffering he had praised'.[15] Regarding an increasingly painful and developing mass as a novel feature of his face (of his being) and as an affliction to bear, Illich lived for twenty years with vigorous honesty about his sufferings and pains and his palliative practises. That he lived as he did, David Cayley reflects, was a significant part of his teaching about suffering for others.

Illich's decision for the mass to remain untreated, even undiagnosed, was a scandal in the broken world. But his 'virtuous performance' of suffering his life, as it was given, 'gave an example and showed a way' different from that which follows after, and is even entrapped by, 'accredited authorities, approved formulas, and diagnostic stereotypes'.[16] Cayley's comments are apropos:

> Illich's unusual way of taking his disease shows the possibility of finding personal meaning in what comes to us and perhaps of regaining a relationship with death as something other than that determined skeletal enemy with whom the doctor wrestles so heroically in the modern imagery of death [...]. Illich's example denormalizes. He proposes no rule about how one should deal with [illness, pain, old age, and dying]. Rather, [...] He fought against "the self-aggrandizing technological myth" that has medicalized the human condition. He fought against the loss of death as a personal act. And, most crucially of all, he demonstrated another way.

Such a demonstration is what the broken world of problems militates against – another way. The world we have manufactured by technological rationalism is a static, stereotyped world. It is the world with problems, only problems, and no answers for the nihilism it conjures except for its familiar repetition of desire and technique. The late modern world, where persons do grow old, do confront illness and do experience pain, suffers life predictably, formulaically and functionally not only risking but also exaggerating experiences of despair that undermine being-in-the-world; or more specifically, being-in-a-situation, experiencing our corporeality and intersubjectivity. Persons conformed to late modern imaginaries, therefore, learn to treat the human condition as yet another problem to protest or to put out, anticipating dissatisfaction, disdain and wishing for death, among other perspectives and actions that obscure and inhibit human flourishing and hope.

Focused further on the experiences of particular persons, one might also find catalysts for resistance in personal narratives that illuminate other exemplars of resistance. You'll recall from Chapter 3, I sat across a table in the early 2000s from a woman who said, without hesitation, 'I am refusing all further treatment. I am going to die'. To add to that introduction, she was a woman participating in a research study and a cancer symptoms management programme at a university clinic where I was working, studying and researching (my interests, at the time, were focused on chemotherapy-induced peripheral neuropathies). I was speaking with her about my research and the ways in which the platinum-based chemotherapeutics she had been treated with were neurotoxic – her peripheral nerves, for example, were experiencing numbness, tingling and pain. But her prognosis was grim. She had a late-stage pancreatic adenocarcinoma with metastases throughout her body. Those of us familiar with her case at the clinic knew she was going to die. But hearing her words was unsettling. She interrupted my silence with the exclamation, 'Let's enjoy our time together!' I found that to be an odd phrase to follow the admission that one is confronting death. But we did.

She requested to remain active within the clinical setting as she had no other family or children – and the university clinic was able to do that (thankfully, we were not beholden to insurance or other forms of payment). She would talk often about her situation: discussing her friendships that have receded during her cancer experience; conversing about her pains and discomforts; acknowledging the accumulating fatigue and distresses that were increasing her dependencies on others. But not all were considered as though solitude, hurt and exhaustion are mere points to dissect and analyse, seeking justification and resolution. And her regular presence in the clinic did not occlude the truth of her loneliness. Her body did not hide the effects of her cancer and cancer treatments. Her eyes, bright but weary, did not hide her anxieties and fears. Yet she remained patient and practised courage. Paradoxically, she remained joyful.

Her joy was contagiously humanising for those in that clinic, where we'd have the opportunity to experience time with her for several weeks before her death. While alone and isolated from so many others, she refused to isolate herself from us at that university clinic. Refusing as such, she gave of herself – revealing the health and sickness of her body, Patricia taught me, at very least, what it might look like to flourish as a human being. She taught me what health and illness of the body might look like even while journeying towards death and refusing with strident conviction the experimental 'hopes' (or 'deceptive expectations'[17]) her oncologists continued to introduce as though magic scissors that might cut out her cancer through trial. (While she endured rounds of treatment previously, an expression of her will to live, she was not sentimental about 'being a fighter' and refused the 'placebo and ritual' of chemotherapeutic hope[18]).

Reflecting on that experience now, I can understand that Patricia's concerns were not on controlling her life and her death as problems. She, as Marcel might suggest, lived throughout the mystery of it all – *together*. But even at that time, while not knowing of the grammar that Marcel provides to our experiences of the human condition, she was a revelation to me; her life catalysed a questioning of modern agency set against problems, preoccupied with *self*-determination and its corollary fetishes for control, that has persisted in my thinking and my work ever since. And I thought about Patricia and modern agency and control and technological rationalities, and of our problematic world, a great deal during that week my mother died.

Sitting vigil, I witnessed the kind of technological schooling that constrains our imagination and disciplines behaviours set towards controlling both pain and suffering, manufacturing meaning accordingly (see Chapter 1). Yet I also witnessed a kind of dance the nurses performed for my mother too. They would draw their faces close to hers and speak all the while knowing the severity of her stroke. The nurses would sing to her as she was being cleaned and changed. They would hold her hand. Brush her hair. Clothe her in beautifully crafted nightgowns, tailored for hospice use. They affirmed her life, ensuring that she would, even in her weakening and withering and unresponsive state, flourish unto death. Their actions were humanising. In the absence of control over her dying, I watched as these persons refused despair and practised care. My mother, and her suffering, was not reducible to a problem to resolve (even if her death rattle and the possibilities of pain were considered as such). She was a person *given* to these nurses for whom they practised their art for no other purpose than to demonstrate love. (And I acknowledged prayerfully all those who have come before, available in their weakness to enable these nurses to practice their art). And I encountered joy, once again, amidst my sorrow, watching these persons, alongside my dad, bear my mother by their bodies; bearing the healthy and sick body of my mother through their touch and tact – resisting, with the art of clinical *care*giving, the problematic life.

Such moral exemplars reintroduce a vision of the world, which many of us have failed to notice. The failure to notice makes sense given the ubiquity and frequency of images and practices, narratives and justifications, which repeat the dogma of particular rationalities incumbent to the broken world. Such experiences do train us to say and to see the world, accordingly; occluding transcendent exigencies which reveal and nurture the human condition, attentive to the realities of being-in-the-world (realities of finitude, if you will). Accordingly, the importance of bodies for re-sourcing hope must be considered. Bodies require attention – against a backdrop and the constant messaging of ideas. Yet bodies summons persons for active responsibility.

The following, therefore, charts towards the conclusion by considering various experiences we might reflect upon while opening up a possibility of living through ageing and dying, differently. Such experiences are the demands of being which we must learn to journey through. The journey is the wayfarer's burden. But the journey is not to be charted in isolation. Rather, bodies (our own and others) summons not only attention but also response, together. We are, by the fact of being, provoked at the start of life to participate in the mystery of being along the way. Such provocations excite the moral life, anchoring it to reality (the object of hope[19]). Such provocations invite a participation in the moral life of virtues, which fosters hope (and a much different kind of hope from that which labours to eliminate [but exaggerates] despair; a hope that incorporates despair[20] and arises within us, as *being*, in communion[21]).

A History of Attending to Bodies

Bodies, who are the persons we encounter in time, remain as such timelessly – persons through memory. And the bodies of the women introduced above, among others introduced previously, remain with me as memories enfleshed in my body, humanising my 'existential judgements'.[22] I can imagine that you all might have such similar memories. But the experience of these bodies, in contact with my own [and my body in contact with itself and the world], have organised, or 'defined and placed', my understanding of existence and of their needs.[23] Without such bodily awareness, without the capacity to feel the world (rather than to *think* the world in abstraction), neither these women nor I would be able to discover a meaningful, rational world – the world 'embodied in me'.[24]

Feeling the world, as such, is the principal fact of being: 'for beyond all experience, there is nothing'.[25] That is to say, only in and through our bodies, our own and in contact with others, might reality as true, actual experience become known. Only by what Gabriel Marcel might regard as incarnate, bodily existence does meaning emerge, realistically – contra the idealism of abstract, primary thought. Such thought, indicative of the broken world, trains persons to become as bystanders who can, by measure and method, accumulate immaterial data and construct worlds of meaning (lessness).

Yet 'our bodies in contact with others' is not to conjure an image where the crude details of our physical, external senses provide all the features we need to have knowledge of another.[26] Although our physical, external senses do matter. And objectively descriptive details are not to be discounted. But such information, if you will, is not received by an 'undefined wasteland' or placed into the 'depths of a forest'.[27] Rather even such objective detail is received into the 'world embodied in me', to circle back to the importance of meaningful, rational discovery. Thus, it is a receptivity caught up into the dialectic of intracorporeal encounters that are dynamic, active and participatory.

The dynamism here is important. If the experiences of an individual become statically pre-eminent, conditioned comparatively to universal generalities and 'stand in for meaningful relationships, or are used as an instrument to gain other possessions, then experiences themselves lose their ability to be meaningful'.[28] Robert Spaemann's 'In defense of anthropomorphism'[29] might offer some complementary explanatory notes here: Spaemann begins his essay raising the question, 'Is this real?' For Spaemann, in ways akin to

Marcel's opposition to primary reflection, an answer to this question cannot be resolved by abstract principles, which descends from the mind to be applied *ab extra* [from the outside]. The world is not a mere constellation of objects upon which questions are asked and answered. Instead, reality is affirmed, faithfully, by the ones asking the question – and by our very existence, we all are asking. Human beings are already caught up into the world in which the answer to the question is assumed. It is assumed as we bear witness to reality. And in a world of correlating persons, we bear witness also to the following, as Spaemann says: 'I see that you are seeing me and talking about me— that what (who) you are affirming is not my body as object, but my self. I am object as subject'.[30] And if that is true for 'I', it must also be true for the other 'I' (Thou) too. Bearing witness to such reality, we must affirm the givenness of other bodies as other persons as our own body is also given. Affirming reality as such, we might recognise 'Persons are real only in plural, that is, as subjectivities that have become objective *for one another*'.[31] For one another, the world might be known, realistically, within each one. (Speamann assumes this paradigm, also 'for every experience of reality'[32]). For one another, we discover a moral realism with meaning.

In that way, attending to others as bodies vitally includes 'a straining [...] towards something' other we might receive, if unshackled of prejudice (i.e. objectifying, functionalising preconceptions).[33] In this way, attending to others as fellow subjectivities includes the experience of that which is transcendent and grants by an inner transformation a new perspective that this other 'embodies *itself* in that human being's acts'.[34] This new perspective is an understanding that comes by way of an irreducible and interpersonal dynamic, which is not only the genesis but also the telos of our being-in-the-world.[35] It is of this latter experience that I am speaking – an experience that includes, simultaneously, both straining commitment (or 'ardour') towards and a 'receptivity' open to encounter.[36] It is an experience that demands participation – a participation that is, enduringly educative and responsively creative.

Let us retreat to experiences with my grandmother: she was agelessly 'old'. At least that was true to my perceptions. My maternal grandmother, the principal and proximate model of old age in my early life, had always presented with white and thinned hair, wrinkled and inelastic skin, measured movements and a frail body – with both arms and hands often bruised from the bumps and knocks incurred while navigating her unsteady world. From 71 to 89, the years of her life that we shared, her body revealed the icon of the so-called fourth age. Although her cognitive capabilities would be the pride of anyone, at any age, she struggled to endure walking distances that steadily decreased over time. She suffered a severe fall in her sixties, from which she never really recovered the healthful *functions* of unencumbered gait.

And through her final two decades, the effort to complete daily activities, including activities of self-care, became increasingly burdensome.

But for much of her later life, Grandma lived alone. Even when she came to live with us (my parents, sister and me), she'd often sit in the 'formal' living room with the nice furniture, away from the action of the home – not wanting to be a burden, distracting the rest of us from our busyness by admitting her frailties. She'd concede as such when we'd enquire, 'Why are you sitting alone?' While I can't say necessarily how others in my family responded, I often accepted her concession and would walk away towards my 'busy' schedule of friends and sport and school – affirming her fears; to remain with her would be burdensome. At other times, the bodily demands of later life did require attention (mine or others) even against her fears.

She eventually moved into a care home, where she would spend her final few years. I'd cycle to her accommodation to visit every so often. I'd find her almost always alone – sitting by herself in her room either working on a crossword or knitting, playing solitaire, or watching her soap operas. (I admit, I shamelessly and thoroughly enjoyed watching these unrealistic and shallow melodramas, while she would knit or as we played cards together). And while visiting each time, for a brief hour or so, I observed her old age.

I found *it* frustrating. As the model of old age in my life, the juxtaposition of her physical frailties and mental vigour, in fact, nurtured a sorrow against her life, which I carried until her death. That she suffered life 'in her body' for so long, I felt was an injustice – an injustice not only for her but also for me, as I did not experience a 'third age' grandparent, like so many of my friends *had*. I thought of her bodily fragilities, her (self-willed and compelled) seclusions and her not wanting to be a burden with pity – contemptuously, even.

I often wondered whether she knew how I thought about her 'problems'. I think she did. But after her death, I didn't revisit those thoughts of pity and contempt for long. And the relief I experienced initially upon her death, which I thought resolved her problematic life, was replaced in time by remembrance. And I have, as time has passed, discovered memories of her interrupting the way I had perceived previously, thinking her later life relative to others (relative to an ideal) as a problem – memories illuminating the ways she engaged patiently with me; for me, even (whether wittingly or otherwise). She was, after all, a real human being. Her life is not reducible to a mere *problem* at all.

I remembered her vividly, for example, four years after her death. I felt the memory anchored into my bones, the first time I shook the hand of a woman whose name I regrettably can't recall (and given my regret, a pseudonym seems deceptive). I shook her hand while working as an intern at a rehabilitation hospital in Mechanicsburg, PA during the final semester of my undergraduate studies. Typically surrounded by peers at my university, and enamoured as I was with the freedoms and fun, the loves and lunacy, of college life, I didn't have or arrange for many occasion to engage with older people. So, the experience of shaking her hand in hospital was distinctive. It was unsettling. It was an awakening experience in many ways – a spark to remember who my grandmother *was* and the ways I had related to and communed with her. In that handshake, memory of my grandmother arose within me and in dialogue – inviting me to think again, to think differently, about later life 'as a problem'.

The patient had suffered a stroke after being hospitalised for heart attack. She was transitioned eventually from acute care and admitted for in-patient rehabilitation where I was working. She was admitted so her physiotherapists and occupational therapists could promote efforts to regain functions of daily living. Similar to my grandmother, she featured various hallmarks of the 'old' old. The memory of my grandmother was complemented by the particularity of this woman's brittle, bony but firm grip; although feeling her hand in mine offered a unique history all its own. And in that particular event, an experience of existential dialogue I've not yet forgotten, I felt the gravity of the work I had taken up – even as a lowly, unpaid intern attempting to earn credits to complete my undergraduate studies.

And that I was tasked with activities that required me to hold and to position and to bear her weight only added to the intense, bodily recollection of my grandmother. We spent just shy of two weeks together, working towards improved functions of gait and upper limb mobility on dry land and in a pool so she might be able to reassert certain independencies. The physiotherapist assigned to her case would brandish these functions of independencies as justification for particular discomforts and distresses induced by the rehabilitation protocols. Such distress, however, proved futile – with little to no improvements gained over those days I knew this woman. And I arrived to work one afternoon to learn that she had died, suffering, this time, a fatal infarction during the night. I reflected on my experiences with Grandma again.

Similar events of remembrance occurred while interning at that hospital and again while working with persons navigating experiences of cancer and cancer treatments during and after graduate schooling in the applied health sciences while in Colorado. Such memories have worked to recuperate an understanding of embodiment and of the human condition our broken world tends to occlude. The recollections are experiences that have nurtured an understanding that we are our bodies; encountering the bodies of others is an encounter with being – their being, a body too. And such encounters have been transformative to understanding the human condition and the moral life as mystery rather than problem.

Such experiences are educative. Over time, I have found it interesting, that memories of one's body do stay with us, raising new questions about their being and ours too.

I find it interesting that the memory of my grandmother's body is that which I recall most vividly when I have shaken hands, held up, or hugged another – not the body she had, as though memory of component parts, but the body she was. You see, when Grandma and I did share occasions to be with each other, we rarely spoke verbally about her old age, her burdens and her struggles. Yet her body, like the hands and body of that woman in hospital, spoke volumes.[37] The demands of bodily life do summons our attention and shape our memory; but the advantages of technique and the promises of control are seductive and can, and often do, dampen our hearing and frustrate the experiences of being-in-the-world. Such modalities stand in our place but do not reciprocate mystery.

Consider this, further: the bodily speech encountered through fleshly, human contact with my grandmother, as her body, is what I had to heed, given the rarity of verbal cues uttered. I had to learn how to pay attention to her as a body. I had to learn how to listen to her as a body when she would come to visit. I continued to learn when she came to live with us and later when I would visit with her at the care home. As I grew older and stronger and more responsible, I had to listen more intently – while supporting the responsible listening modelled by others. But I can't say that my learning to listen was sufficient. It certainly was not.

Nevertheless, even failing to be as attentive as Grandma might have needed, my experience with her was learning of how to observe the body; repeating what I said above, not as something she merely had, but as the body she was – even if I was an unwitting and poor-minded student of such learning for quite some time; until well-after after her death, in fact.

I had to learn to be attentive to the efforts required to move, to the bruising on her arms and legs (from bumps, scrapes and tumbles) and to the crescendo of creaking and crepitus. I had to learn to be attentive to her as a body, which included, in part, the physical words of burden she did actively share with us. If I didn't learn well enough during her later life, Grandma, through memory, did and continues to set me towards an understanding (rather, towards the necessary *sense*) of others, in the fullness of their corporeality – the reality of their bodily being. In this way, mysteriously, she remains 'at once present and gone forever [...] but a veiled questioner with whom [I] may still carry on a dialogue'.[38] And this is important; had she not actively shared herself with me, even as burden self-perceptions persisted, no such dialogue would have been initiated.

Such dialogue might be that which has provoked necessary *sense* of sympathy. It could be that my sensing memory of Grandma's physical words, if you will, in a continuing dialogue has helped to relieve abstracted ignorance of later life, which depicts control, independence and absolute agency over both life and dying as functional ideals required to succeed along with the depredations of corporeality as objective problems to fear and to resolve by technique.

Through continued questioning and dialogue, I no longer pity or disdain. Rather, I remember joyfully; thankfully – for such memories have been essential to understanding the human condition as it is lived, realistically.

Put differently, I do remember with vivid sympathy (viz. understanding) that which and of whom I had often touched and, thus, have been touched by – giving my grandmother aid to walk her to or from a room any way I could, to guide the weight of her body as she would rise or sit (and to catch her when unstable) by whatever means available to me, or to embrace her with love (and to be embraced by love), feeling every bone and the fragility of her skeletal frame. By such tactility, by the presence of her as a body alongside me as a body, I was sensitised to corporeality – I was sensitized to her humanity. And, responsively, I was (unwittingly) humanised too.

'To touch and to be touched', as Richard Kearney has commented, 'is to be *connected* with others in a way that opens us up. Flesh is open hearted'.[39] It opens us to hope.

Bearing the weight of others, embracing others, we learn to feel *with* and to experience difference, to encounter another, intimately. We also discover the mutable peculiarities of reality that demand our moral attention and decisive action. Touch, in the way that bears others, as I have learned from these women identified above, 'brings us into intimate contact with […] [and] expresses body and soul at once'.[40] This is why it is humanising.

It is by such active inter-corporeal 'contact' that we are humanised, respectively, and situated to moral realism. Humanised realistically, as such, one begins to discriminate against inhumanity and the ideals of unreality – learning to recognise life-in-the-world, which is not reducible to problems that need to and can be fixed to suit an ideal. Of course, such understanding comes with time and with an ongoing participation with and for the lives of others. Such understanding is shaped by an education one receives in contact, or in participatory conversation with others – learning to be attentive to and responsible for concrete, particular bodily life.

Certainly, Marcel's moral realism has helped to elevate the experiences of bodily life, both noble and ignoble, healthy and sickly, youthful and aged, living and dying. Marcel depicts an education through our bodies, elevating the experience of bodily life as a kind of carnal hermeneutics, not too dissimilar to that described by Richard Kearney. Kearney too seeks to elevate bodily life where '*Yo veo con las yemas de mis dedos/lo que palpan mis ojos* [I see with my fingers/what my eyes feel]'.[41] In learning to be attentive to concrete human life, or concrete life more broadly (including the lives of flora and fauna, for example), one can be drawn beyond the contours of a broken world and the icons of its fragmenting static functions while learning to journey towards and through a world where hope is enfleshed – where the peculiarities of human life and human frailties and where the actualities that cultivate despair summons a humanising touch, calling for the vicariously responsible action.

Touching Real Life, Becoming Responsible

Responsibility grounds hope, realistically: One needs to *be* ready to express concern, to love and to act responsibly *for* another when despair threatens the human condition. And despair often does. One needs to be ready, whether sick or well, cared for or carer, old or young. To be ready, however, one must *become* as those with 'taste and tact': 'Touching well is living well. Hermeneutics begins there, in the flesh'.[42] For is it by such *touching* that we might learn and be strengthened to bare (to reveal) and bear (to carry) the burdens of human life, together.

Such a hermeneutic, however, *depends* on being attentive to the experience of 'dependence'. This includes an understanding of dependence as an experience of our corporeality, which includes the recognition that others are needed essentially and not instrumentally to make/to practice our sense of the world. But also understanding acknowledges the reality that others are also dependent. Being 'dependent' and attentive to 'dependence' requires practice. Such practice strengthens us against a potent modern narrative history and incumbent social performance (as illumined by accusative burdens) that consider particular meanings of independence (i.e. self-sufficiency, individual choice and control) as dogma.

And the practice of dependence is realistic. That is to say, the human condition is fundamentally intercorporeal; thus, interdependence is basic to the human condition. Unfortunately, we are trained to think otherwise – prioritising independence while coming to regard dependence as seen with both transitive and accusative burden as an unwanted or feared state of being.

To understand otherwise, to observe the dignity of dependence, is to learn again that the human condition is not reflected in the imagery and ideals of self-sufficient demigods with capacity to overcome ageing and death. We must learn again by *touching reality*, acknowledging through the drama of the ethical life that persons, including ourselves, are dependent on a network of complex relations where touching well might be humanising: 'It is not the isolated individual but the responsible person who [...] [sic] truly *live*'.[43] Attending to such reality, to the practice of responsible interdependence, this humanising network of inter-relating and contingent persons over time can excite an understanding where dependence is experienced as a strength instead of as undesirable fodder for despair.[44]

Let's consider health, again, as an example: Karl Barth has argued health is a corporate phenomenon – making the claim that when one person is ill, all of society is ill.[45] Such a claim is not illusory, but conditioned by his understanding of human being as irreducibly relational. Accordingly, when one cannot exercise the practices essential to will for health by their own strength, another may, and therefore must, bear such practices on her behalf – providing due care where one is otherwise weakened by the depredations of age or illness. And so on and so forth. The sociality of practising the will for health, together, even when inundated by the forerunners of death, frailty and disease, ensures that the one *and* the other can flourish *as human beings* – both the sick and the well, bearing the coinhering health and sickness of their bodies, bare their respective and correlating humanity. Human dignity is understood through moments of such dependence and not reified or held in some state of high-flying, idealised competence, status or rationality.[46]

Rather, dignity is discovered in the practices of *being* that overcome the habits of *having*, as persons come to acknowledge reality and accept the frailty, weakness and death of human finitude – in such acknowledgement and acceptance 'lies the germ of solidity and a new kind of power which consists of the creativity typical of [...] being'[47] – and specifically, of being together, wayfaring along the way 'through an overgrown field'[48]; performing the hard, tragic work of finitude. Such work is possible, however, through love – such work is anchored, realistically, by fraternity – by the freedom one experiences before an 'other', similarities and dissimilarities fully acknowledged.[49]

Such work, carried out in responsible communities of correlating persons, performs the mutual dependence one has with another. Such habitual work is humanising. The practice of such receptive correlation throughout one's life stages, readies each one particular person to give and to receive due care, and thus, the capacities, or rather virtues, to relate as one to her fellows in both healthfulness and sickness, in youth and in later life – readying us to bear the burdens of our fellows, *gratefully*.

Put differently, the activity of the moral life, in many ways, includes the practice of and reflection on receptivity. Marcel suggests the experience of 'Gratitude implies above all an intense awareness of our own receptivity'.[50] The practice of receptivity, or our experience of gratitude, shapes our being. It opens us up towards others. Rather, as Marcel continues:

It unites us with the others outside of us, whom we consider the source of this feeling. I purposely used the term "source," rather than "cause," and "feeling" rather than "relation," for gratitude is an act of sympathy, not a mechanical relation, and a feeling always transcends the relationship which produces it. [...] Gratitude, however, is not just of the moment. It persists, it is rooted in memory, it is memory.

But receptivity, in order to be(come) memory, must be practised. That is to say, if gratitude, awareness and receptivity correspond to memory, we must learn to recognise a particular 'other' as the vital source of such memory. Such recognition deepens our understanding (our necessary sense) of otherness and the fullness of corporeality.

In this way, gratitude extends from the phenomena of another's living and it excites response – after all, gratitude is an activity of the moral life. The response must, therefore, reflect the value of the incarnate source of the gratitude. It must attend to the bodily demand such receptivity understands, while turning towards the experiences of the other's flourishing. To put it plainly, consonant with a familiar Matthean pericope, gratitude clothes, feeds, comforts, cares and so on – it performs these actions according to need (the claim the other makes upon us). It too bears the gravity of old age and of dying for those whose strength for life is weakened by depredation and disease; but who stand no less as the source of my being (and I theirs). Accordingly, in an ever-widening circle of humanising sociality, gratitude illuminates and strengthens community – its very activity, community-life, shapes intercorporeal receptivity as a realistic phenomenon that is humanising.

The Practice of Availability

The possibility of receptivity depends on acknowledgement – or what might be considered availability. Before I say anything further about availability, let us consider the current experiences of persons in our present age: as Louise Aronson admits, reflecting on a patient for whom she makes house calls, 'I can, and do, write prescriptions for Dot's many medical problems, but I have little offer for the two conditions that dominate her days: loneliness and disability.'[51] Of course there are others who do provide care and attention. But what is given is 'not enough'.

Not only is it not enough, but these other caregivers have ageing bodies and incumbent strains too. Some might even be dying (or hugging their own death, anticipating suicide[52]).

Haider Warraich details such strains among carers in his book *Modern Death*.[53] We must attend to such strains that reflexively burden us and our fellows. Such attention, however, must not become a repetition of the kinds of self-nouns (i.e. self-sufficiency, self-control, self-determination, etc.) a modern anthropology champions but extended, merely, to one's family or narrow circle of caregivers (as though a family is but an analogue of the individual, repeating a familiar phrase, 'We will take care of our own') – risk for overwhelming despair persists in such situations; as caregivers suffer their own experiences of burden, the care for the other's body demanding attention also suffers while the aims of a modern agency, that is, burdenlessness, prove aimless.

It is for this reason that Warraich reminds his reader, for example, 'One in four American adults provide informal caregiving at any moment. [...] the overwhelming majority of caregivers are female, and 85 percent of them are related to the patient. [...] Caregivers suffer not only in resources but also in health: [...] experience[ing] increased rates of depression, anxiety, and insomnia and an increased risk of suicide'.[54] Warraich continues, 'despite being so intimately plugged into the [healthcare] system, too many times they [caregivers] are so invested in the well-being of another that they forget about themselves. But perhaps the greater problem is not that caregivers are ignoring their healthcare, but that healthcare ignores caregivers'.[55]

Knowing this failure of the system to persist, physicians and nurses might despair (as Warraich does) that they will have no legal recourse to 'address their [caregivers'] needs unless they also happen to be a patient'.[56] Of course, they could, at the very least, enquire with due concern and attention to the other, seeking to know how such caregivers are doing – a small act of compassion that might help another to bear a burden. (Meryl Comer reflected on the twenty years of caring for her husband who suffered from dementia, with only one particular physician asking her about her well-being: 'When you have a disease that always wins no matter what one does, you need someone to make you feel what you are doing matters'[57]).

But what does Dot (and do her carers) need? 'What she needs', as Aronson continues, 'is *someone* who is always there, who can help with the everyday tasks she now finds so challenging, and someone who will listen and smile and hold her hand'.[58] But no *one* person can execute such functions. Aronson knows this too; yet a robot caregiver can.

Aronson is quite considered on her conclusion. And for those who might object to a robot caregiver, Aronson offers her retort: human beings do not necessarily provide care for others. Some, in fact, can excite particular distress (not to mention experience caregiver burden and distress too, as concerned Warraich). At times, while intending well, human caregivers can do harm, even execute 'wilful acts of negligence and abuse'.[59] Robots, programmed for caring, can mitigate such damages. And her challenge to critics of a technological solution to the crises of 'not enough' care extends further: the introduction of robot caregivers needs not to replace but should supplement human caregiving, which, at present (in the US), is a sector of vocational work or volunteerism that remains underserviced – a looming workforce crisis.

To be sure, Aronson, a celebrated geriatrician and professor of medicine, will understand well the demands required to attend to these problems. She appreciates that it might be best if Dot would have an army of caregivers. Yet Dot does not have such an army – she has a daughter and friends and a telephone support network. A robot could be a suitable solution to the problem of 'not enough' care. It is certainly a solution that fits the consumer model of successful ageing; that follows with economic rationalities that find in such solutions a labour force to celebrate; and the increasing reliance persons have on technological artefacts to carry out daily functions. But as well-meaning as I would argue Aronson is, the problematic life persists in such thinking – functional solutions to functional problems. The principal role for Dot to play in the solution being introduced in this discussion on technology in Aronson's *Elderhood*, is the agent consumer who desires for (or objectively has) particular functional needs to be met. That she might benefit from owning (or leasing) such a robot is surely possible (even probable) – technologies most often do deliver on their aims[60] – but such a possession cannot practice gratitude, for example. Such robot caregivers, and sadly even some human caregivers in a late modern marketplace where *useful unemployment*[61] is a fiction, can only be had, used, and used up. Such functional entities cannot correlate with Dot, becoming hope.

Well, to be sure, wherever there is a person, 'true companionship *can* be created'.[62] The reason being, such persons are not robots – or tables and chairs, as Marcel has discussed. Wherever one sets a table, a chair, a robot, or a mobile phone, 'I do not make any difference to [it]'.[63] It is simply there to be used for a given purpose; these objects that remain external to me can come and go, be exchanged or moved. And they remain unaffected by their relation to other things or me; save for forces of use or misuse can cause material damage or wear. But this does not matter to the object either. Such objects do not experience the world. That is not true of relationships where 'the preposition *with* properly applies' – Marcel is adamant, such a preposition does not apply to the objective world. This is not true of relationship where I might be in relation *with* Thou (an 'other' immersed in her subjectivity); 'where my relationship *with* you makes a difference to both of us'.[64] Persons, while degraded by the broken world, are not obliged to it.

And Aronson herself is not beholden to the problematical. In fact, in reading Aronson's important book, one gathers a sense that she is an -ician in the true sense of the Hygieian tradition of medicine.[65] Like all grateful -icians who attend to patients as 'water carriers, [and] bearers of responsibility', as Seamus O'Mahony describes (opposed to the -ologist who is preoccupied with the problems of cause and cure),[66] Aronson assumes clinical responsibility for her patients, like Dot, and grieves over the 'not enough'. She is also not like the 'state nurse' who Gabriel Marcel describes as 'a functionary to the marrow of her bones; she has failed to realize that to look after a sick person is something that goes beyond everything that can be defined as a function'[67] – certainly a realisation a robot could not apprehend. For Aronson, relationship *with* her patients makes a difference to both her and them.

Accordingly, I trust she would appreciate Marcel's concerns regarding the *value* of caregiving and the distinctions he makes between problems and mysteries. But 'Value', centred on the practice of gratitude, 'can only be incarnate—it must be lived. As soon as we are tempted to objectify it, we disembody it, we strip it of its authenticity'.[68] The robotic resolution to the problem of caregiving would, and does (when considering current systems of labour and the market metaphors that discipline the technique of work), do just this.[69] Yet that does not mean technologies do not have a place – one must, however, be attentive to ensure that technologies of any kind, industrial, digital, political, or moral, do not work against the formation of the person, or a society of persons, while obstructing their fulfilment.[70]

To become attentive in this way, one must be(come) open to encounter the other – to be interrupted by the incarnate *value* of otherness, which we only discover when living with and for others along the way. Where gratitude excites a feeling that one is gifted with the presence of another, availability habituates an openness – or readiness – for such gratitude.

But availability is a virtue under-practised in a late modern world. As argued in Chapter 3, for example, the triumph of autonomy and the alienation of persons towards self-determination and self-control marks the characteristics of a late modern anthropology. For ageing persons, the priority of independence continues to persist as an ideal to strive towards. The results of such thinking: as Age UK reports, 58% of the 3.8 million older adults living alone are 75 years or older. And those persons living alone in later life are more likely to require emergent care, live with multiple comorbidities and experience mental health conditions.[71] And loneliness persists as a principal cause of suffering for persons.[72] Of course, loneliness is not simply experienced when persons are alone – there are many factors and occasions that contribute to experiences of loneliness. It is, however, 'the social equivalent of physical pain, hunger, and thirst'.[73] Loneliness evidences the need for sociality, as the absence of such intercorporeal connections is physically insufferable.[74] Loneliness reveals an exigent need, which the illusion of independence works to occlude.

But, as discussed throughout, persons conformed to a broken world become increasingly familiar with functional explanations of human experiences, which are known fully by technological categories and rationalities. They are introduced as evidence for our knowing *how* the body works. Moreover, by the powers of the problematical, persons become (or are encouraged to become) self-sufficient (encouraged to habituate pride, a vice).[75] A vice which turns persons ever inward, but without a corporeal centre of our being, which finds its source in sociality.

But sociality (social *life*) cannot be instrumentalised, for such thin social bonds (which we often go along with) are mediated by technique and position the other as mere a cog in social machinery, which does not bare life: 'People meet, or more accurately, bump into each other. That makes quite a racket. [...] But there's no center, no life, anywhere'.[76]

By principle (i.e. late modern autonomy and pre-eminence of independence as a policy aim) the late modern anthropology isolates the individual from her fellows, both Divine and human, and erects as essential the self-determinism that, in the end, cultivates despair while masquerading as hope. The self-sufficient and solitary icon of the Heraclean archetype in the preceding chapters seems exactly is fitting – similarly, the modern individual is encouraged by policy, practice, programme and posture to be as an 'independent' freed *from* all others (related only through functionalised relations, like those of consumers and providers).

Marcel, in turn, denounces such malforming principles and programmes, including the ethics, policies and practices that call persons to adjudicate the moral milieu where life is lived in the midst of death but without particular, incarnate attention to those fellows who gather and claim us for mutual recognition and cooperation at the nexus of intracorporeal crises. Such claims, however, are as the divine claim that secures the freedom, meaning permissions, to become who we are (human beings), in communion with our fellows, both near and distant. Karl Barth rightly articulates the realism of such claims: they are clothed, as Christ, in the 'garment of another' who stands before us as the one to, with and for whom life is to be lived.[77] (Such claims, of course, return our attention to Matthew 25, as discussed above).

In particular, incarnate attention, our responsiveness to bodily burdens (our own and others), demands the consideration of an individual person's essence – to one's bodily nature. After all, as Bonhoeffer contends, reflecting on a theological anthropology, 'a human being *is* a human body'.[78] This means, then, that 'A human being does not "have" a body or "have" a soul; instead a human being "is" body and soul.'[79] Thus when the body is speaking through its aches and pains, whether acute or chronic, our very nature is calling out for attention, baring a particular moral reality of an individual person – that a body demands attention, claims others' attention as well.[80]

That is to say, the revelations of an ageing or dying body and the incumbent strains experienced by particular persons ought to be given attention, not only by these individual persons themselves (if possible) but also by both domestic and qualified carers, from spouses, partners and children, to nurses and physicians, among other health professionals and volunteers. Rather than being a source of transitive burden, however, the gaze by others ought to be considered differently. Others ought to learn to listen to the claims and respond accordingly – gratefully; it is the way to understand reality and the moral life of being-in-the-world.

The Responsible Action of Bearing Burdens

Listening to and for reality must be performed amidst (even against) the whirring acceleration[81] of instrumental reasoning and the crescendo of individualist autonomy, which tend towards the bodies of the ill and infirmed as objects to control (or who don't attend at all, leaving persons 'independently' responsible for their successes in later life). Such listening must be performed with a readiness to adjudicate and to advocate good (clinical and familial and neighbourly) caregiving, which might be described as the 'due care for those who cannot provide care for themselves [...] [and] ever-vigilant to concentrate upon [each] *demanding* body'.[82] And truly, no one person can *care* for themselves either. (Even self-love, theologically (i.e. Matthew 22:37–40), is caught up by a logic of sociality – love of God and love of neighbour). So, with 'gratitude and responsibility, we must [...] take seriously the historicity and particularity of embodied human beings struggling *together* amidst the ambiguities of present crises and towards the flourishing of human life even unto death'.[83]

The work of receptivity and gratitude, the practice of availability, is a social initiative where attention to the demands of bodily life, to the baring of human corporeality (viz. inter-corporeality), must become a bearing together. For the Christian, bearing overcomes inhumanity. But such bearing is not only humanising for the Christian – life together is essential for being human, in general. In fact, as Dietrich Bonhoeffer contends (a sentiment not discordant to Marcel either), 'Only as a burden is the other really a brother or sister and not just an object to be controlled'.[84] Because that is true, universally, it is also true of the Christian. It is for that reason Bonhoeffer can say, 'Christians *must* bear the burden of one another'.[85]

Bearing others' burdens, we bare humanity – the humanity of our fellows and our own. For the Christian, baring humanity, we become as icons of the humanity of God ('who suffered and endured human beings in the body of Jesus Christ. [...] as a mother carries her child, as a shepherd the lost lamb. [...] In suffering and enduring human beings, God maintained community with them').[86] And such an understanding of bearing is significant for our discussions encountered in this book. Only through the experience of corporate bearing, might persons, together (believers, half-believers and non-believers, alike), be enabled to protest a programme of techno-capital means introduced by a healthcare marketplace committed to maintain a distance between one and one's fellows as idealised policies of independence, medicalised rationalities and functional hopes prioritise a kind of static description of successful ageing and good dying according to a late modern orthodoxy (a broken world) against the actualities of real life – of finite, mortal, intercorporeality and mutual, fleshly dependence. (And the preceding, breathlessly long sentence is important too – it carries a cadence and urgency that you'd see in my voice and which I trust you might hear on the page).

That the sounds and slogans of the bodies of many particular persons in later life, ageing and dying, summons others to the 'structure of responsible life' in a society offers evidence for the kind of ethics that Bonhoeffer and Marcel advocate while opposing others where functions and problems of various kinds persist. But focusing on Bonhoeffer's *Stellvertretung* (vicarious representative action), such ethics becomes 'most evident in those relationships in which a person is literally required to act on behalf of others'.[87] Refusing such action, such bearing, when required, is to foreswear humanity. Or, as Bonhoeffer contends, theologically, it is to 'deny the law of Christ'.[88] It is to deny the love for your neighbour and obstruct her advantage. It is a vanity, which runs (drawing our attention, once again, to that important epigraph).

Digging in through the encounter, acting in the service of others, loving and seeking the advantage of others, means to 'stand in their place. [...] incorporat[ing] the selves of several people in his own self'.[89] Such standing in one's place is what it means to bear another (or with Marcelian vernacular, to be *available* for another – a characteristic of being we will take up further below).

Of course, Bonhoeffer's reflections on Christology, his study of Jesus Christ, orient his understanding of bearing.[90] Yet he gives examples of fathers as well as statesmen and instructors to offer sociological confirmation of his claims in this regard. He also turns to medical professionals to give example. Regarding a father (or mother or guardian to be more exacting), he 'acts on behalf of his children by working, providing, intervening, struggling and suffering for them. In so doing, he really stands in their place'.[91] Any attempt by this father to live as though he were an isolated individual, independent of others, especially his children, 'is a denial of the fact that he is actually responsible' – a responsibility, like all others, which he cannot altogether escape.[92] 'Fatherhood', as Marcel might chime in dialogue, 'only exists as the carrying out of a responsibility, shouldered and sustained' (degenerating when delimited by mere, specific functions of role).[93]

Such a moral vision of responsibility reflects a shared rather than individualistic agency implicit in Bonhoeffer's understanding of human beings. Bonhoeffer's reflections on the social phenomenon of friendship might offer some insight. The character of friendship is marked by *vicarious representative action* as an interceding for one another. Such intercession and self-offering are to be understood and practised as need-determined, mutual and non-competitive – expressed by a self-implicating and concrete correlation.[94] While several examples Bonhoeffer provides to exemplify *vicarious representative action* are often rich in power relations and risk patriarchy, the relation of ageing persons to partners, peers, kin and other carers might correspond better to friendship marked by mutual responsibility, even if asymmetrical due to frailty or illness. Moreover, *vicarious representative action* as friendship must also be conformed to an understanding of freedom, which might 'release others from all [one's] attempts to control, coerce, and dominate them with [one's] love'.[95] Such friendship, as such, is not a self-centred and unmediated exercise of dominance over another but an attentive exchange where correlating persons ('equal in our inequality', as Marcel would stress[96]) are taught and enabled, by a mediated encounter with Christ in and for the world, to disclose their needs, desires, sins and ideations so that each might learn not only to attend to such disclosure out of love but also to situate the vocation of friendship where fidelity for the well-being of each other might be promised (and practised).

Devoting oneself to the flourishing of another, often many others, in this way is vicarious representative action. Such devotion anchors and bolsters friendships, but not only friendships. Consider, for example, the medical professional. The concrete case of a physician and a patient introduces a relationship where the responsibility of the physician to give due care for the benefit of the patient is obvious. But the physician is not responsible only to the patient. She is responsible to many patients and to the whole of the profession, for which she executes her service. Only then might she fulfil her vocation.[97] Accordingly, as a physician she 'must recognize and fulfill my concrete responsibility as a physician no longer only at a patient's bedside, but, for example, in taking a public stance against a measure that poses a threat to medical science, or human life, or science in general'.[98] Any attempt of the physician to abandon her responsibilities through their denial, or a 'myopic self-limitation', is careless and negligent.[99]

But devotion to one's real responsibilities, thus to those for whom one is claimed to exercise responsibility (bearing), is the vocation of human beings. Devotion (availability), therefore, to the flourishing of those for whom one exercises responsibility is not a devotion to acquire idealized abstractions or to secure particular objects of a so-called good. Instead, such devotion is to 'the affirmation of human beings and their reality'.[100] Bonhoeffer, continues saying, 'Action in accordance with Christ is in accord with reality because it allows the world to be world and reckons with the world as world, while never forgetting that the world is loved, judged, and reconciled in Jesus Christ by God. [...] No one is commissioned to leap over the world and turn it into the kingdom of God'.[101]

Thus, to act accordingly, to be responsible, is to attend to real (bodily and disclosed) needs rather than abstracted desires or projections. One is to become responsible to the '*domain of concrete responsibility*'.[102] And concretely, to be sure, there is no escaping the other.

She is, and they are, in the particularity of being *Thou*, the occasion for persons to exercise humanity and to be humanised in accord. Vicarious representative action is concrete is this way. 'The attention of responsible people', therefore, as Bonhoeffer contends, 'is directed to concrete neighbors in their concrete reality. Their behavior is not fixed in advance once and for all by a principle, but develops together with the given situation'.[103] Developing together, the aim is not towards an unrealistic ideal or disincarnated 'absolute good' (like independence, which seems reified in successful ageing campaigns and policy statements), but to act meaningfully '*in accord with reality [das Wirklichkeitsgemäße]*'.[104] Neither ideal nor policy but reality bares, or reveals and constitutes, the truth and limits of our responsible human action (of our bearing).

Bonhoeffer's ethics of responsibility echo Marcel's schooling, which assumes, in the first instance, that particular phenomena are real. He assumes persons *are* experiencing subjects who are involved (immersed) in life – whose being is as a becoming on a journey through the exigencies (tragic, transcendent and otherwise) of being. This is Marcel's starting point.

For our purposes, it is thus important to posit the depredations and dependencies, pains and perturbations that frailty or disease render, and which we experience as our bodies, *are* real. Not only real but also significant. Like hunger and thirst, like the will to move, like the need to love (and be loved), we experience such urgent demands as others do too. Moreover, we *can* work to assess and analyse such reality. But such work must remain as reason disciplined by reality – as reason that is 'material, inductive and unsystematic'.[105] Such reasoning is thus reflective; or, following Marcel, our experiences of reality are dialectically ambulatory, demanding reflective movements between life and thought along the way. Establishing his dialectic in his *Metaphysical Journal*,[106] Marcel argues that such reflective practices limit abstractions and permit a particular interaction or tension between life and thought that refuses a flattening out of either. Accordingly, to encounter Marcel through both his philosophical writings and to encounter others (and their lives) introduced through his plays is to discover in conversation a reflective practice that labours to work 'up from life to thought and then down from thought to life again, so that [one] may try to throw more light upon life'.[107] For Marcel, the work is as a mapping out of human life as it is lived concretely rather than an exercise of delimiting abstractions 'in the high void of "pure thought"'.[108]

For our present task, I have attempted such reflection – drawing upon experiences with ageing and dying as well as pain and suffering, which both I and others have experienced or I have experienced with others. The concrete experiences of person ageing and dying, as with those persons giving care (whether familiar, professional, or otherwise), and the words (by both bodily and verbal speech) that give expression to such experiences, have served as the topography from which and to which the present task has laboured to map. And, I think, this work of existential cartography, if you will, reflects the way we might *together* begin to understand the human condition – in the depths, breadths and heights of being-in-the-world, but also, with critical ire, human 'being' reduced by both rationalist and idealist fabrications. Such cartography involves a wayfarers' journey over and through the sorrow and joys, tragedies and triumphs of human life, without prejudice and without the need to discover meaning beyond the meaning that is *a* human life (and *a* human community).

That I have emphasised 'together' is vitally important: the ontological connection we share with others, the very real experiences of touch and being touched, so to speak, is what establishes the possibility to flourish as particular human beings. This too requires, as Donald MacKinnon has summarised, a reflective learning that 'we are through our relationships with other people; we acquire in a common life the concepts through which we bring home to ourselves what our experience is'.[109] MacKinnon goes on to say this of Marcel's philosophy of being: 'There is no initial privacy from which we go out to meet the world. Rather the private is something that draws its very shape from the public life by which it is nurtured.'[110]

That is to say, we practice our personal existence together with other persons in public. For Marcel, ontological existence is necessarily bound to being in relation: 'existence takes on the character of including others'.[111] Put differently, 'When I am bound to the other in love, I am'.[112] Perhaps it better to conclude, 'We are', for both I and Thou are ontologically nurtured in the correlating encounter. Such immersion into intersubjectivity, into being together, is not unique to Marcel. One can see such anthropology summarised by Karl Barth's dictum, *Ich bin indem du Bist*, which means I am by the fact that you are.[113] It is an expression of being, which one discovers also in several African anthropologies of relational being, which build from Ubuntu philosophies/theologies where an understanding of the human condition is thoroughly relational and participatory.[114] Thus, the human condition is a creation of intersubjectivity: 'We create each other and need to sustain this *otherness* creation. And if we belong to each other, we participate in our creations: *we are because you are, and since you are, definitely I am.*'[115]

Sharing perspectives, Marcel echoes: existence is not to be thought as self-centred. The problem of being is not for one to determine as though an independent – 'the idea of an individualist, monadistic, and self-contained self is an illusion that must be dispelled'.[116] Thus, Marcel's anthropology is not an idealism. It is rooted by his realism; accordingly attentive to the bodily demands of being-in-relation corresponds. That is to say, Marcel's realistic account acknowledges the presence of *otherness* within the world of being we are immersed. Rather, mere acknowledgement is not adequate. Responding to the other, whose summons is as a call to being, must be basic to our understanding of being-in-a-situation. Other persons situate our being as one who is called by an 'other'. Thus, 'To be is to be for the other.'[117]

Accordingly, the private, that is, our own unique experiences, our peculiar subjectivity, draws its strength from such public life too. This private–public interface is something Marcel learned from American idealist Josiah Royce[118] and retained as he developed his realism contra idealism: 'What Marcel learned from Royce was a continuing sense of human societies as enduring spiritual communities from whom individuals could, and indeed must, derive not only their elementary human formation but also a kind of interior strength powerful enough to sustain them in periods of personal disintegration and catastrophe.'[119]

The derivation for Marcel, you can likely expect at this point, was not from a unifying thought (or abstract ideal) but from the experiences or concrete presence of one with and for another. That I might consider it good or right or just to offer aid to a person that needs to cross a road is one thing. It is entirely different to be available and to give aid actively when exigencies demand a response. The latter action re-sources such interior strength in both parties. The former does not need anyone else, at all, to be self-congratulatory.

It is by way of concrete experience (through the urgent demands of being both one's own and corporate, or communal) that the derivation of this private–public interface is discovered. And only through such communion (public) might individuals find hope, enfleshed (private) – only then might persons, in community, responding rationally (thus realistically) to the urgent demands of the human condition, and each of our peculiarities of being, discover the dignity of hope (in oneself and for others) regardless the status of one's healthy and sick life.

'Regardless' is a challenging perspective to maintain, however. The readiness to be attentive, to encounter others with gratitude and to be available for them, however, does not come by the way of rational assent or efficient technique. Such virtues must be habituated by both discipline (use) and time (repetition). And because virtues, like medicines taken for our well-being are dose dependent, such availability must correspond with the practice of fidelity – especially when *the way* does not bring with it a promise of escape from despair.

Hope Enfleshed and Strengthened by the Practices of Fidelity

Communion is humanising: Availability, parallel to the earlier discussions about responsibility, is a demand of being, we discover, for example, when we accept the physical demands of a frail grandparent when she walks from a room to a garden seeking fresh air and the warmth of the sun. To be available to give of oneself for help is a humanising act for both persons; requiring, of both correlating persons, admission of weakness, dependence and mutuality. To be available in this way for my late grandmother (and she for me), was a gift Id did not acknowledge until well after her death. That I experience and reflect upon being available to others in remembrance, encountering others and acting responsibly for their claim on me too, is also a gift, for which I am grateful.

Receiving the will to movement from another, such that we might responsibly receive bodily weakness with ours strengthens both, enabling movement for a person burdened by the depredations of ageing is indicative of being. Sharing such burden is humanising. And so too is the act of waiting with another who is sickly or who is dying, as we did for my mother. Sitting vigil is the humanising action of being available – and such availability is certainly not passive. Such demand requires attentiveness and endurance, through which persons might exercise creativity that nurtures communion, reviving the human condition from the degradations of the problematic world – even amidst the hardships of living, ageing and dying which are real, and often unrelenting. Such communion opposes the static positioning of a neutral observer who is enabled by method and model to stand dispassionately adjacent to her situation and others, who stands nowhere, while observing worlds with illusions of objectivity, disciplined by 'a metaphysics of abstractions, deductions, and dialectical speculations'.[120] Yet such communion must be strengthened for it to endure both tragedy and triumph and the ongoing pressures of despair that petition for escape.

The practice of fidelity is thus necessary: where the practice of responsible presence (or availability) 'makes room for another person in myself'[121] (meaning in my experience of being), the practice of fidelity strengthens the attachment. It is a virtue, which 'can create, heal, and sustain broken human connections'[122] through the freedom of being to receive and to be available for another. And as we read in Chapter 2, broken human connection can occur as individuals confront the burdens that threaten to isolate and demean them, while living through the frailties of later life. Fidelity, however, admits burden outright, but refuses withdrawal – not with static constancy, but creative commitment.

To be sure, we can know 'Fidelity truly exists only when it defies absence, when it triumphs over absence, and in particular, over the absence which we hold to be—mistakenly no doubt—absolute, and which we call death.'[123] I experience such fidelity each time I remember the women I have discussed in this book – for such persons, like others you might remember, continue to 'live in us' and remain as the other (Thou) 'with whom we may still carry on a dialogue'.[124] Accordingly, the practice of fidelity anchors communities of caring through the promise of active and ongoing gratitude, which transcends time (by way of memory). But it is a practice that 'can only be shown to a person, never at all to a notion or an ideal',[125] which ensures the feeling of gratitude (memory) is duly responsive to who and what is being communicated by the other. As such, fidelity requires ignorance too.

Discipline, time and *ignorance* are conditions of the practice of fidelity. Ignorance is the 'fundamental' rejection of the kinds of optimistic ends that functional hoping stereotypes into its rationalities and ethics. It is also a rejection of the 'idea' of another I might have within a circle of my mind that precludes genuine encounter. Thus, ignorance is a rejection of the functionalist, problematical disposition towards human life. 'In swearing fidelity to a person', as Marcel explains, 'I do not know what future awaits us or even, in a sense, what person he will be tomorrow; the very fact of my not knowing is what gives worth and weight to my promise.'[126] Not knowing, practising ignorance, therefore, energises the practice of openness, for I must ask again and again, moment by moment, day by day, who it is that stands before me and through whom I must hear the claim of her body upon mine in its momentary particularity and possible difference.

Fundamentally ignorant, refusing stereotyped response accordingly, fidelity accepts fragility and finitude experienced by persons, it does not forget the experiences of suffering and despair are real and mutable. Such acceptance is practised, continuing as presence, 'whatever the circumstance may bring'.[127] 'Whatever the circumstances' is not an expression of apathy – a lack of caring. It is an expression of endurance – no matter what might come, I will remain with you and for you – even through death.

Such ignorance, such endurance, is the condition upon which one's practices of fidelity can be renewed, creatively. That is to say, fidelity nurtures, along with availability, a perspective that the moral life, inclusive of conditions of despair, demands a humanising touch, which recognises the essence of dignity grounded by the frailties of corporeality and of the participatory actualities of human being that is indissolubly and non-reductively relational – contra technical.

Relational rather than technical means that one must be readied to accept a particular inefficiency. Patience is thus needed. And it is patience, a virtue that habituates fidelity, which binds each of us to each other through not only joys but also sorrows.

Let me explain. Patience, as a corollary practice of fidelity, is not passive. Patience is active. But like all virtues, it is not beholden to the broken world which observes patience as passivity (a vice), waiting for particular ends to arrive as though a commodity that comes from a specific, even stereotyped, technological intervention. Patience does not wait for the 'good death' to be acquired for them through medical means or through the maintenance of particular ideals. Such passivity, as we have seen previously, fosters the kind of hope that is but despair in disguise and remains with such hope(lessness).

We should be dissenting from such passivity. The ethical life enables such dissent of the kinds of imaginaries that have only a single answer to the challenges that persist in human life, including pain and suffering, old age and disease (the answer: all challenges are but mere problems to resolve by the administration of human desires through techniques and incumbent rationalities). Of course, this does not mean that the practice of patience encourages belligerence over new findings and methods of pain management, caregiving, or medical- and psychotherapies that attend to the sufferer, whether ageing or dying. We mustn't mistake a critique of the broken world, and its stereotyped commitment to technique, with the creative agency of medical and surgical and palliative interventions, for example.

Neither does it mean that one ought not to lament the pain and suffering experienced by persons in the world – or wait for such pains and sufferings to become filled with meaning. Both of these responses would be indicative of suffocating inactivity. And I've already said that patience is active.

Accordingly, patience (habituating fidelity) requires the practice of courage also. Courage 'consists primarily in facing something'.[128] The resolve it habituates is not free from fears. It is not free from concern that fidelity might be rejected and availability abused. It is certainly not free of those fears that accompany reflections and encounters with death, including its forerunners, old age and disease. The one who is courageous does not deceive 'oneself about a given situation. It [Courage] reaches its zenith, on the contrary, when the situation is most clearly appreciated'.[129] In fact, the practice of courage requires such appreciation in order to discern well how to respond rightly to the (changing) situation. (Patricia, e.g., was courageous to confront her death joyfully. Yet courage was exercised differently earlier in her cancer experience where rounds of chemotherapeutic trail were endured). But courage is also an act of denial – a refusal to accept our anxieties (and thus the expectations of our desires and fears) as final. Such denial bravely unmasks the masquerades of despair, exposing it to the light of reality. (Patricia too, demanding our time, sharing her life with us, performed such an act).

Courage practised, as an accompaniment to the virtues introduced thus far, might strengthen the stamina of one (whether that one is being cared for or doing the caring) to abide in caregiving without accomplishments, for example, and to continue to practice the creativity of fidelity (finding new ways to remain available and responsibly grateful). Courage is in no way beholden to static instrumentality.

The palliative caregivers who attended to my mother embodied such virtues – excellences demonstrated daily. While particular actions remained coupled to the narrative of control and manipulation (as discussed in Chapter 1), this was not the only narrative being performed. Their collective efforts demonstrated a way of saying and of seeing the world that is able both to accept and to protest the grievous actualities of pain and suffering. Having received my mother, their work was disciplined by both patience and courage, and narrated through their bodily practices a vision of medical caregiving that worked 'with the body's capacity to both flourish and languish',[130] and charts a moral space where grief could be expressed and where all of us at my mother's beside were enabled to receive her as the one for whom we might practice 'that profound courtesy',[131] love.

The Christian tradition has understood this courtesy to be true (although many Christians have not always remained faithful to its practice). Understanding as such, participating *in situ*, in the situation of our being-in-the-world, we discover (with Christ, for the Christian) the true beginning and end, the true character, of hope.

And hope loves. Yet love, which orients us towards the heights and depths of being, as the above practices bear witness, is not easy. But its *work* is located by the recognition of each other's weakness and inability to control life as a problem. Love is a mystery; immersive and not instrumental. Love holds on to others; through such embrace the human being discovers transcendence. Rather than hugging death as All Calamity (as the closed fate of being enslaved by time), which persons attempt to acquire power over, love is free from the captivity, which tempts to death.[132] Free, it is not bound to particular methods of overcoming or ensconced by particular aspirations. Free, it is not exempt from disappointment and depredation. Free, love finds its meaning when persons practice being-for-others, keeping hope alive within the depths of one's being too.[133] In this way love *expands* the space where persons might flourish as human beings, even unto death.

It opens up the world: Henri Gourier offered a response to Marcel's play *Le Monde cassé* [The Broken World] for *L'Europe Nouvelle* (20 January 1934).[134] 'Underlying the four acts', Gourier concludes his review, 'there is the question that goes beyond all pragmatisms: what does it mean "to exist?".'[135] And he turns then to praise Marcel for the philosophical value of his realism, explaining with due discernment the distinction between problem and mystery, which we've been exploring throughout this short book:

> If one always situates a problem in front on *oneself*, the problem of being can never be posed, because I can never detach myself from being in order to take my distance from it. Gabriel Marcel calls 'mystery' that inability to be reduced to a '*problem*'. However, to say that being is a *mystery* is not a way to close off inquiry or debate; on the contrary, we must explore where it is, and that is not interior to a concept, nor interior to an intuition—no knowledge can circumscribe being; rather, it is being that holds all knowledge. I attain it when my attention, reflecting back upon itself in recollection, feels its existence stirring to a naked consciousness.
>
> Then a world opens [...].[136]

The practice of fidelity, among the many immersive practices above, stirs such consciousness, which 'engenders a sense of hope'.[137] Hope emerges as an expression of the human condition and discovers that death, like life, is no problem at all. Rather, through our participation (our 'sharing of fellow-feeling'[138]), immersed in the mystery of being, we might discover 'death does not have the final say and that there is an inexhaustible realm of being which transcends death and the problematic world' of ageing and dying, frailty and finitude.[139]

Practising Hope, Wayfaring Through Despair

Frailty and finitude have oriented a discussion throughout that interrogates the broken world and the kind of technological habits that have become commonplace as both question and response to the problematic life. But, as the conversation evolved above, bodily demands, which old age and dying certainly introduce, summons a humanising touch, which recognises the essence of dignity grounded by the frailties of corporeality and of the participatory actualities of human being that is indissolubly and non-reductively relational – contra technical. Only through such participation, immersed in being for our fellows, might we learn to live hopefully through despair, together, even when despair persists. Only through such participation might we act rightly – moment by moment (responding to the particularity and mutability of personal experiences) – with and for each other, discovering ontological strength through our admissions of weakness, need and mutuality. This is the wayfarers' journey.

Reflecting on both Bonhoeffer and Marcel, among other sympathetic voices and experiences above, we charted the learning and moral response that remains attentive to the journey through concrete human life. Such learning and moral realism draw persons back from the contours of a broken world, and the icons of its fragmenting static functions, while wayfaring towards and by walking through a world where hope is enfleshed – where the peculiarities of human life and human frailties and the actualities that cultivate despair summons a humanising *touch*. Reflecting on such responsible practices, we learn of hope resourced (recuperated[140]) to illuminate life along the way while resisting despair and humanising the problematic life.

Put differently, this final chapter encourages resistance against the late modern preoccupations and instrumental instantiations that have conformed particular idea(l)s that are indicative of the broken world – the world that over-prioritises the problematical. Such a world, as diagnosed, renders persons ageing and dying, experiencing pains and suffering, for example, vulnerable to despair while flattening out the moral life and demeaning the human condition. Of course, resistance doesn't come by way of an efficient technique manufactured and commodified for use. Discovering resistance doesn't come by way of having a solution to a problem. Such ways are a capitulation to repeat the logic of a broken world.

Positively, however, we are invited to reflect on and to experience another way; summoned to give our attention to the artful drama of human lives, which we might recognise in the lives of others *and* experience within ourselves (both simultaneously). Attentive to such drama – to the realism of the human condition – we might encounter despair and joy, tragedy and triumph. But we will also discover the opportunities to practice patience, courage, presence and love, for example, so that such virtues might be(come) enfleshed and persons, including ourselves, might flourish as responsible fellows and hopeful friends even when problems go unresolved (while experiencing frailty and finitude, ageing and dying) in a late modern age.

Hope is, therefore, not an instrumental phenomenon, which functions as a commodified aim for which particular strategies and stereotyped techniques might secure – but can't because such aims are as ideals that hang ineffectually in the air, without touching the actualities of corporeal life. The illusion of perpetual independence is one such malformed hope, as we discussed. So too is the promise of escape from the threat of the kind of death we do not want (i.e. the uncontrolled death).

Resourcing hope, we are thus set towards the task of discovering its ontological ground, its source in being, which is discovered through the dialectic of living and reflection. Hope, sourced as such, is a realistic hope – a humanising hope experienced 'from the inside' (situated in the world alongside our fellows). Our discovery, or understanding, of hope and the moral life of being is acknowledged and realised through our immersion in the world and our experiences of it, including the depths of despair, while learning to be(come) attentive to the complexities and ambiguities of reality. Such immersion must be grounded by intersubjectivity – our attention alerted to the quirks of personal experience and with the awareness that the human condition as irreducibly relational. And reciprocally, wayfaring alongside each particular other we might encounter is grounded by the fact of 'being-in-a-situation' – positioned by 'the exigencies' or demands of being that are both peculiar (to each individual person) and binding (summoning a communion of persons).[141]

For our corporeal life *together*, hope is not resolved by technique but grounded by touch. And such touch, as I have implied already, is disciplined by a range of practices and their repetitions over time; experiences which resource the human condition to see and to embrace the needs of another, to bear them and they us (regardless of the condition of the healthy and sick life of one's body). Hope, as such, is a humanising 'activity of the moral life' opposed to the problematic life of a broken world.[142]

To be sure, a broken world constructs a civilization 'from the outside' but fails to maintain an understanding of being 'from the inside' for those struggling for life and towards death. A broken world habituates a way of seeing *things* and interprets the experiences of functional loss, reduced sense of self and agency, and fear of burden, discomfort and the like, as well as the actualities incumbent to disease and disorder, without any teleological vision – a broken world with its functionalising metaphors, instrumentalizing reasoning and objectifying desires resources despair with no hope at all.

Connected with such despair are some institutions, policies, programmes and professionals who offer metastasising endorsements, that affirm life as wholly disposable and utterly unworthy of existence in particular present (or possible future) states. Such endorsements deny being, smothering the dignity of finitude and occluding mutual recognition and cooperation, regardless of the state of health or sickness one might be in.

Resisting such despair, the activity of the moral life *hopes to and for one another over time*. Such hope endures. Such hope excites critical reflection and provokes a questioning of despair and (functional) hoping in a broken world such that one might not die in flight from despair; and, thus, captive to it.

We ought not to want such a death. We ought not to want such a life, even if the illusions of dignity, of control and of benefit are presented with the full support of clinical best practice and legal precedence. We ought not to want the narratives that bolster such postures that risk despair and its masquerades without learning to live through despair – without learning to live life in the midst of death.

Yet we ought not to want to frustrate continued progress in clinical measures and competent care when people are confronted with the limits of human life either. Rather, we ought to be reflecting discerningly and creatively about a response *for* persons ageing and dying in a broken world. We ought also to reflect again and again about what it means to flourish as a human being, even unto death by medical means and the provision of care executed by the helping professions. As above, we must continue to reflect repeatedly and creatively about how one might die hopefully, even while wayfaring through despair.

We should and we must.

The condition here is that hope is not a commodity or an abstraction that risks despair while offering illusions of flight from it – as though one has a choice to make. Rather, the condition is that hope is practised as a virtue caught up by an intersubjective and reflective pedagogy that forges a readiness to confront despair, ageing and death – a pedagogy that recovers a strength for *being*, while living *and* dying. Hope is habituated and enfleshed as person labour to listen and to hear 'the stories of forbearers who learned how to go on when it wasn't clear there was a way to go on'.[143] Such listening and hearing can become the foundation of hopeful communities that learn to endure together – who learn to participate in the cultivation of hope, in the possibility of its virtue, as it is offered through the performance of mutual recognition and commitment.[144]

Such hope precludes the sort of narratives that seek to evade death and escape despair. Such hope precludes narratives that elevate the efficient decision of the solitary and self-sufficient hero and acknowledges that one 'cannot hope alone'.[145] Such hope precludes narratives of stereotyped agency and technological rationalities that persists in our modern milieu. Such hope 'faces difficulty in a creative way by learning to improvise'.[146] Such improvisation might also cultivate or correspond to courage, for example, which not only 'names' that for which we are determined (exigencies of being) but also enables us 'to see them through' – albeit, perhaps, and quite importantly, *differently* than imagined in the first instance.[147] Such hope learns not only from our encounter with others but also from those stories of the Christian scriptures and traditions, from 'stories of Israel and the Jews [that teach us] [...] to live in a world in which we aren't in control'.[148]

Such encounter with others, while received with gratitude, is as invitations to give of our attention and to follow; they elaborate and epitomize the way of hope in and through the darker situation of life. Hope, as with other virtues, enfleshed in the lives of those whose habituations make them concrete, can confront such times decisively – making decisions, not at a crossroads of choice, but because of whom such persons have become; because 'they could have done nothing other than what they have done'.[149]

Resourcing hope as such might interrupt the familiar narratives of hope-as-commodity in a broken world, revealing them to be as a profane doctrine, which torments, tendering despair as it promises respite. Such understanding might discipline our being and ready each one of us for the long struggle amidst present ambiguities and trials, while seeking ways to practice availability, responsibility and fidelity that is hope-enabling – performing hope as a material and social practice that cultivates the strength of *being*, recuperating hope in others, for others, degraded by a broken world.

Enabled to grow and to develop hopefully, we might understand the freedom of the human condition, and its dignity, which endures through the triumphs and tragedies, if not also the calamities and comedies of our finite and frail existence. Such hope can sustain us even during times of prolonged darkness and imminent death, which the anxieties of ageing and disease can excite. Yet hope does not determine such sustain as though an idol. Rather, hope is freedom that opens us to the realities of the world (of being-in-a-situation) and liberates us to pursue human beings, that is, to become what and who one is, through living and dying.

Notes

1 Hernandez, *Marcel's Ethics of Hope*, 5.
2 Robert Spaemann, 'In defense of anthropomorphism', in *A Robert Spaemann Reader: Philosophical Essays on Nature, God, & the Human Person*, eds./trans. D.C. Schindler and Jeanne Heffernan Schindler (Oxford: Oxford University Press, 2015), 77–96 (88–89).
3 A note written by a fifty-year-old man from Massachusetts (Etkind, *Or Not to Be*, 13).
4 As introduced by Friedrich Nietzsche in the first chapter: See Nietzsche, *Will to Power*, 22.
5 Van Wijngaarden, et al., 'Reading to give up on life', 257–264. See also Els J van Wijngaarden, Carlo J W Leget and Anne Goossensen, 'Till death do us part: The lived experience of an elderly couple who chose to end their lives by spousal self-euthanasia', *The Gerontologist* 56, no. 6 (2016): 1062–1071.
6 A fifty-two-year-old woman suffering from multiple sclerosis penned this letter. Her husband was jailed for several months for assisting her suicide (Etkind, *Or Not to Be*, 101). For Vivien Sleight, the possibility that we might be able to secure freedom from further unwanted torment through both decision and opportunity to die is what confers hope for those confronting hopelessness (Sleight, 'Hope and despair', 354).

7 See Marcel's discussion about 'corporeity' in his 27 March 1931 entry in 'A metaphysical diary': Marcel, *Being and Having*, 81–83.

8 'The fact that despair is possible is the central datum here' (Ibid., 104).

9 For an anniversary review of Illich's *Medical Nemesis*, see Seamus O'Mahony 'Medical Nemesis 40 years on: The enduring legacy of Ivan Illich', *The Journal of the Royal College of Physicians of Edinburgh* 46, no. 2 (2016): 134–139.

10 To gather a sense of Illich and the kind of intellectual, religious and social experiences and encounters that gave shape to his life and thought, see George Cyr, *An analysis and evaluation of Ivan Illich's social and educational philosophy in the light of his early development and the major critiques of his theories*, PhD Thesis in McGill University, Montreal (not published), 1990, 6–32: https://escholarship.mcgill.ca/concern/theses/0k225c187.

11 David Cayley, *Ivan Illich: An Intellectual Journey* (University Park: Pennsylvania State University Press, 2021), 443.

12 See Gabriel Marcel's discussion about the techniques of degradation here, Marcel, *Man Against Mass Society*, 27–56.

13 Ivan Illich, *Limits to Medicine: Medical Nemesis: The Expropriation of Health* (London and New York: Marion Boyars, 1976), 166. Emphasis is mine.

14 Ibid., 166.

15 Cayley, *Ivan Illich*, 444.

16 Ibid., 447.

17 Referring here to the 'hope' contained in Pandora's pithos, as introduced in the introduction (Franco Montanari, Chr. Tsagalis and Antonios Rengakos, eds., *Brill's Companion to Hesiod* (Leiden: Brill, 2009), 77).

18 Seamus O'Mahony, *The Way We Die Now* (London: Head of Zeus, 2016), 172. Patricia would surely have made Seamus O'Mahony proud. O'Mahony is a confessed 'oncology apostate' and refuses with Illichean force the technocracy and 'false hopes' incumbent in his profession, medicine, from which he has recently retired his clinical practice (170). His writings are worth reading, as seen in snapshot throughout this book.

19 Hernandez, *Marcel's Ethics of Hope*, 60.

20 Ibid., 62.

21 Marcel, *Homo Viator*, 52.

22 Marcel, *Being and Having*, 10.

23 Ibid., 10.

24 Ibid., 115.

25 Marcel, *Mystery of Being (1)*, 47.

26 Ibid., 49.

27 Ibid., 118.

28 Hernandez, *Marcel's Ethics of Hope*, 59.

29 Spaemann, 'In defense of anthropomorphism', 77–96.

30 Ibid., 81.

31 Ibid., 83.

32 Ibid., 85.

33 Marcel, *Mystery of Being (1)*, 47.

34 Ibid., 48.

35 Spaemann, 'In defense of anthropomorphism', 77–96.

36 Marcel, *Mystery of Being (1)*, 56.

37 Richard Kearney, 'Carnal hermeneutics', in *Imagination Now: A Richard Kearney Reader*, ed. M. E. Littlejohn (London: Rowman & Littlefield, 2020), 99–119 (99).

38 Marcel, *Creative Fidelity*, 150.

39 Kearney, 'Carnal hermeneutics', 104.

40 Ibid., 105; c.f. Jean-Louis Chrétien, 'Body and touch', in *The Call and the Response* (New York: Fordham University Press, 2008), 83–131 (85).

41 A phrase from Mexican poet Octavio Paz's *Este Lado* [This Side]: Octavio Paz, 'Este Lado', in *Árbol adentro* (Barcelona: Seix Barral, 1987), 33. Richard Kearney refers similarly to Paz, as cited by Jean-Lois Chrétien in his *The Call and Response*, suggesting 'Touch fosters a synesthetic community of sensing. Or, […] "I touch you with my eyes/I watch you with my hands/I see with my fingertips what my eyes touch"' (Kearney, 'Carnal hermeneutics', 106).

42 Ibid., 100.

43 Dietrich Bonhoeffer, *Ethics*, vol. 6, trans. Reinhard Krauss, Charles C. West and Douglas W. Stott; ed. Clifford J Green, Dietrich Bonhoeffer Works (Minneapolis: Fortress, 2005), 258–259.

44 c.f., Stephen Wright, 'When dignity', *Nursing Standard*, 19, no. 33 (2005): 30–31.

45 Barth, *Church Dogmatics*, III/4, 324–397.

46 As Marián Palenčár reminder her reader, Marcel regards such 'dignity' as *'decorative'*, ornamental and stilted (Palenčár, 'Marcel and human dignity', 123).

47 Ibid., 124–125.

48 Ibid., 120.

49 Ibid., 126.

50 Gabriel Marcel, 'The concept of spiritual heritage', Confluence: An International Forum 2, no. 3 (1953): 3–15 (4).

51 Aronson, *Elderhood*, 301.

52 Marcel, *Being and Having*, 104.

53 See the discussions about caregiver burden in Haider Warraich, *Modern Death: How Medicine Changed the End of Life* (London: Duckworth Overlook, 2017), 171–190.

54 Ibid., 178–179.

55 Ibid., 179.

56 Ibid., 179.

57 Ibid., 180–181.

58 Aronson, *Elderhood*, 301.

59 Ibid., 303–304.

60 Hartmut Rosa discusses such optomised caregiving by robots in Japan, where research has positively portrayed their usage. However, Rosa critically evaluates the happiness or gratitude expressed by the users, writing, 'with the robots' help, [the sick and old] are released from an alienating situation that is severely awkward and uncomfortable for them. In a culture in which bodily processes and odors are perceived as something extremely embarrassing that should be concealed at all costs, and in which it is considered immoral to be a burden to others, requiring any sort of care represents an existentially alienating experience. Robots' performance of the necessary tasks in this situation in place of human beings may not yield any resonant encounters, but it does render merely indifferent what was previously an outright repulsive relationship to the world' (Harmust Rosa, *The Uncontrollability of the World*, trans. James C. Wagner (Cambridge: Polity, 2020), 83).

61 For Ivan Illich, useful unemployment refers to those situations where people are valuable to themselves and others but detached from corporate-controlled commodities and services. For an introduction to such discussions, see Ivan Illich,

The Right to Useful Unemployment and Its Professional Enemies (London: Marion Boyars, 1978), 7–16.

62 Marcel, *Mystery of Being (1)*, 180. Emphasis is mine. Such companionship is certainly not guaranteed—we are not dealing with a certain commodity of a given technique.

63 Ibid., 181.

64 Ibid.

65 Seamus O'Mahony, *The Ministry of Bodies* (London: Head of Zeus, 2021), 38–40.

66 Ibid., 39.

67 Marcel, *Mystery of Being (II)*, 39.

68 Marcel, 'Spiritual heritage,' 12.

69 I encourage you to read Illich on shadow work or on disabling professions. Read also George Ritzer's *The McDonaldization of Society: An Investigation into the Changing Character of Contemporary Life* (Thousand Oaks: Pine Forge, 1993); *The McDonaldization of Society in the Digital Age*, 9th edn. (Los Angeles: Sage, 2018).

70 Moyse, *Art of Living*, 131–161.

71 See the AgeUK 'Later life in the United Kingdom 2019' fact sheet. Available here: https://www.ageuk.org.uk/globalassets/age-uk/documents/reports-and-publications/later_life_uk_factsheet.pdf

72 Lars Andersson, 'Loneliness research and interventions: A review of the literature', *Aging and Mental Health 2, no. 4* (1998): 264–274.

73 Louise C Hawkley and John T Cacioppo, 'Loneliness matters: A theoretical and empirical review of consequences and mechanisms', *Annals of Behavioral Medicine* 40, no. 2 (2010): 218–227 (219).

74 See John T Cacioppe and William Patrick, *Loneliness: Human Nature and the Need for Social Connection* (New York: W.W. Norton, 2008).

75 Marcel, 'Ontological mystery', 31.

76 These words shared by Christiane highlight the dis-ease incumbent to Marcel's *Le Monde cassé* (Marcel, 'The Broken World', Act I, 46–47).

77 Barth, *Church Dogmatics*, III/2, 584.

78 Dietrich Bonhoeffer, *Creation and Fall: A Theological Exposition of Genesis 1–3*, vol. 3, trans. Douglas Stephen Bax, ed. John W de Gruchy, Dietrich Bonhoeffer Works (Minneapolis: Fortress 2004), 76. Emphasis is mine.

79 Ibid., 77.

80 Ashley John Moyse, 'Responsibility for the broken body: Exploring the invitation to respond to the presence of the other', in *Treating the Body in Medicine and Religion: Jewish, Christian, and Islamic perspectives* (London: Routledge, 2019), 17–28.

81 By 'acceleration' I am reminded of Hartmut Rosa's important book, *Social Acceleration* where he considers, in part, the technological-technical acceleration of late modernity, which has changed the perceptions people have of time and space, as well as of social relations, cultivating a risk for particular ethical and socio-political challenges like those taken up in this book. See, for example, Rosa's discussion of technological-technical acceleration, Hartmut Rosa, *Social Acceleration: A New Theory of Modernity*, trans. Jonathan Trejo-Mathys (New York: Columbia University Press, 2013), 97–107.

82 Ibid., 26

83 Ibid.

84 Dietrich Bonhoeffer, *Life Together; Prayerbook of the Bible*, vol. 5, trans. Daniel W Bloesch and James H Burtness, ed. Geffrey B Kelly, Dietrich Bonhoeffer Works (Minneapolis: Fortress, 1996), 100.

85 Ibid. Emphasis is mine.
86 Ibid., 100–101.
87 Bonhoeffer, *Ethics*, 257.
88 Bonhoeffer, *Life Together*, 101.
89 Bonhoeffer, *Ethics*, 258.
90 Bonhoeffer, *Creation and Fall*, 213–224.
91 Bonhoeffer, *Ethics*, 258.
92 Ibid., 158.
93 Marcel, *Homo Viator*, 109.
94 David S. Robinson, 'Peccatorum Communio: Intercession in Bonhoeffer's use of Hegel', *Studies in Christian Ethics* 28, no. 1 (2015): 86–100.
95 Bonhoeffer, *Life Together*, 44.
96 Palenčár, 'Marcel and human dignity', 126.
97 Bonhoeffer, *Ethics*, 293.
98 Ibid., 293.
99 Ibid.
100 Ibid., 262.
101 Ibid., 264, 267.
102 Ibid., 276.
103 Ibid., 261.
104 Ibid.
105 Philip Mester, 'Gabriel Marcel: Mystery of being', *Dominicana* 48, no. 2 (1963): 129–136 (130).
106 Marcel's philosophy of dialectical reflection, if you will, emerged initially in his *Journal métaphysique* (1927) (Gabriel Marcel, *Metaphysical Journal*, trans. Bernard Wall (London: Rockliffe, 1952).
107 Marcel, *Mystery of Being* (1), 41.
108 Ibid., 41.
109 Donald MacKinnon, 'Drama and memory (1984)', in *Philosophy and the Burden of Theological Honesty: A Donald MacKinnon Reader*, ed. John C McDowell (London: T&T Clark, 2011), 181–188 (185).
110 Ibid., 185.
111 Marcel, *Mystery of Being (II)*, 33.
112 Zachary Willcutt, 'Marcel and Augustine on immortality: The nothingness of the self and the exteriorization of love as the way to eternity', *Marcel Studies* 5, no. 1 (2020): 1–18 (14).
113 Barth, *Church Dogmatics*, III/2, 248; see also Moyse, 'Responsibility', 18–20.
114 Desmond Tutu, *No Future without Forgiveness* (London: Rider, 1999), 34–46.
115 Michael Onyebuchi Eze, 'Ubuntu: Toward a new public discourse', in *Intellectual History in Contemporary South Africa* (London: Palgrave MacMillan, 2016), 181–192 (191).
116 Cheng-Ling Yu, 'Hope and despar: A discussion on the atheistic existentialist, evolutionary biologistic and intersubjective accounts of hope', *Marcel Studies* 5, no. 1 (2020): 19–36 (30).
117 Willcutt, 'Marcel and Augustin on immortality', 14.
118 The influence of Royce on Marcel can be seen, for example, in a series of articles Marcel prepared for *Revue de Métaphysique et de Morale* (1917–1918). The essays were published late (1945) in *La métaphysique de Royce*.

119 MacKinnon, 'Drama and memory', 182.

120 Mester, 'Marcel', 130.

121 Hernandez, *Marcel's Ethics of Hope*, 91.

122 Ibid., 88.

123 Marcel, *Creative Fidelity*, 152.

124 Ibid., 149–150.

125 Marcel, *Being and Having*, 96.

126 Ibid., 47.

127 Marcel, *Creative Fidelity*, 154.

128 Marcel, *Mystery of Being (II)*, 159.

129 Ibid., 159.

130 Autumn Alcott Ridenour, 'Suffering, death, and the significance of presence', in *Treating the Body in Medicine and Religion: Jewish, Christian, and Islamic Perspectives*, eds. John J Fitzgerald and Ashley John Moyse (London: Routledge, 2019), 184–196 (190).

131 Richard Selzer, *The Exact Location of the Soul: New and Selected Essays* (New York: Picador, 2001), 80; c.f. Ridenour, 'Suffering', 190–194; Moyse, 'Responsibility', 25–26.

132 Joseph Godfrey, *A Philosophy of Human Hope* (Dordrecht: Martinus Nijhoff, 1987), 104–108.

133 Marcel, *Mystery of Being (II)*, 160–161.

134 Henry Gourier, 'Henri Gourier's critique in *L'Europe Nouvelle, 20 janvier 1934*', in *Gabriel Marcel's Perspectives on the Broken World*, ed. Katherine R. Hanley (Milwaukee: Marquette University Press, 1998), 153–158.

135 Ibid., 157.

136 Ibid., 158.

137 Lisowski, 'Speaking of mystery', 21.

138 Albert Randall, *The Mystery of Hope in the Philosophy of Gabriel Marcel* (Lewiston: Edwin Mellon, 1992), 345.

139 Lisowski, 'Speaking of mystery', 21.

140 Marcel, *Mystery of Being (1)*, 83.

141 Mester, 'Gabriel Marcel', 129–130.

142 Hernandez, *Marcel's Ethics*, 114.

143 Stanley Hauerwas, *The Character of Virtue: Letters to a Godson* (Grand Rapids: Eerdmans, 2018), 97.

144 Hernandez, *Marcel's Ethics*, 58–73.

145 Hauerwas, *Character of Virtue*, 97.

146 Ibid., 97.

147 Ibid., 113.

148 Ibid., 97.

149 Ibid., 187.

AFTERWORD

The care of vulnerable patients is for sale to the highest bidder and the one who technologises the process most innovatively reaps the greatest profit. Or so it seems.

Why are the first three-quarters of this wonderful little book so difficult for me to read? Because as a practising physician, they ring true. Too true. And they ring tragic, perhaps, in the way John Donne describes funeral tolling. For whom does the bell toll? Donne asks. Who has died? Why, the care of the sick and dying, of course. We have chased the sacred out of those practices. Ashley Moyse seeks to restore it.

In my mind I divide the book into two parts: Chapter 4 and everything else. If 'everything else' is the diagnosis, Chapter 4 is the antidote and a potent one at that. Jeffrey Bishop says, 'diagnosis is easy; therapy is difficult'.[1] Therefore, before we get ahead of ourselves and consider the merits of Moyse's treatment, let's consider briefly the diagnosis articulated in the 'everything else'.

Modern medical practice prizes certainty and exactitude. That which can be measured has value and status. She is in stage IV kidney failure, but the kidney function is a bit better today, we doctors say. Or: the tumour, a hepatocellular carcinoma, shrunk by 2 mm. It is by contrast difficult to articulate the depth of a physician's compassion or the profundity of her integrity, so we elect to discuss kidney function and tumour size over compassion and integrity. The latter sounds nice on patient brochures and hospital advertising schema. But the virtues rarely feature in formal teaching during daily rounds on the medical wards.

Valuing the measurable means that functional, technological solutions will necessarily attract the greatest attention. If a pill or procedure can improve nutritional status, let's pursue it. We can measure nutritional status by checking bloodwork. A registered dietician can count the calories a patient consumes. We can prescribe an appetite stimulant. If that fails, we can place a nasogastric tube. If that fails, we can attempt total parenteral nutrition through a fancy sort of intravenous line. If that fails, we can place a percutaneous gastrostomy tube through the wall of the stomach and directly pump in liquid nutrition. Never mind that grandmother eats when her family visits and spoon-feeds her. Never mind that the only metric hospitals and care homes monitor with regard to spoon-feeding is the number of hours staff are detracted from doing other more 'valuable' tasks. As Moyse suggests, technology instrumentalises knowing for the purpose of doing. If there's a technological fix, we in healthcare opt for it.

But this creates a conundrum. Biomedicine lacks a framework for making sense of unsolvable problems. By *unsolvable* I don't mean problems lying in wait of a fix. I mean problems for which no solution will exist before the patient dies. What, for example, are we doctors to do with incurable cancer, or advanced Alzheimer's disease, or the patient who is fully dependent on all activities of daily living? What is the *point?* Such solution-less problems are largely disvalued in medical practice. The patient for whom no fix is possible ceases to receive the attention of the army of specialists who earlier staved off death. The patient is handed over to those end-of-life experts who will manage his symptoms and socialise until he's dead.

Moyse says that unsolvable problems in a broken world create meaning-lessness, and meaninglessness foments despair. Those who despair feel that they are simply waiting around to die. Why not, then, take control and hasten death? Why not die by suicide, or, better yet, sanitise the process by electing euthanasia? For the patient whose problem is unsolvable, physician-assisted suicide and euthanasia charm and seduce. They promise control over dying and offer a rational medical fix.

This is Moyse's diagnosis as I see it. And he's on the mark. If he misses something, it's that although the *culture* of medicine functions according to a certain technological rationality, there remain individuals within every branch of medicine who actively resist this cultural pull. Indeed, there exist healthcare professionals – albeit few, perhaps – throughout medicine who strive to practice the very virtues that Moyse commends. But their number is too few, and Moyse knows this.

His Chapter 4, then, is a clarion call to healthcare practitioners and others to re-sacralise care of the sick and dying, and his method is to expand upon the remnant who practice virtuously by practising the virtues. Attention, responsibility, availability, burden-bearing, friendship, gratitude, fidelity, patience, courage and love – when practised over time – create the conditions necessary *not* for eliminating despair but for incorporating despair into a kind of robust hope.

Reading this book, I could not help but think of a friend of mine – a former patient, actually – who is well into the fourth age. Most of his friends are dead, and his children and grandchildren live at a distance. We started having intermittent lunches years ago as his spouse's health was deteriorating. He needed to get out of the house and talk to someone, and I was one of the few people still around. In time, he got to know my family. He invited us around to his house for coffee or brunch; we invited him to Christmas dinner.

He was nearly 98 when his spouse died. Despite an initial outpouring of sympathy from those who knew her, the calls and cards quickly dried up. While re-reading Chapter 4, I found myself wondering about his loneliness and my own ability to be available, my own capacity to be a burden bearer. How much can I give amidst competing demands from my busy medical career and family? And what about fidelity? Moyse says fidelity admits burden outright but refuses withdrawal. I would like to believe that I will refuse withdrawal, that I will exercise patience. But now it is easy to be a friend to him; his health is spectacular. What happens when he declines and attending to him feels burdensome? Will I be available then? It takes one type of courage to pledge fidelity to blood relatives or professional clients; it is quite another to remain a faithful presence when no one expects you to show up and showing up itself is drudgery. Faithful, courageous friendship, then, is a mystery.

The thread of mystery weaves throughout Moyse's book. If we relate to the sick, vulnerable, isolated and ancient not as problems to be solved but as mysteries to be engaged, despair is mitigated. On this side of perfection, despair can never be fully eliminated; it persists in constant tension with hope. But by regarding others as mysteries, they become sources of endless meaning. I'm partial to the way Emmanuel Levinas puts it. He says the 'Face of the Other' summons us, overflowing our preformed conceptions.[2] The person we thought was a finite being, we come to see as infinite. This is mystery: a person of infinite depth, of infinite meaning. Where meaning inheres, hope prevails.

This book inspires me to wonder how different society would look where each of us to 'adopt' one or two others whose bodies and/or minds are failing, who need friendship or spoon-feeding or love. I live in a city of about 8 million people, where 1 in 8 is over the age of 65. Could we seven-eighths befriend and attend to the one-eighth? Some people may find the thought of it easy – virtues of fidelity, availability, responsibility, friendship and love come naturally to them. But for many more of us, habituating to availability and responsibility for lonely or dying people takes practice over time. Moreover, while the work of caring faithfully for another is not measurable in the same way as kidney function, it is good work. It is ennobling and humanising work. Indeed, such work is *sacred* work.

In a society where the healthy or younger commit to caring faithfully for the sick or older, care of the vulnerable cannot be commodified and sold to the highest bidder. To be sure, there are costs incurred – time, sweat, sacrifice – but the return on this investment for both a caregiver and care receiver is far greater than either can calculate. It prompts a reordering of loves and a reprioritising of the urgent. Attending to the bodies and souls of others forces us outside ourselves. It causes us to see through blurry lenses and navigate the world with cautious steps and motorised wheels. Pledging fidelity towards another restrains our own self-indulgence. And there is always someone sicker and older, which means in due course, each of us becomes caregiver and care receiver.

So much of this life reinforces the values of independence and self-sufficiency. Moyse calls us to lay it all down and instead to open our eyes to the mystery of the other.

Lydia S. Dugdale
Dorothy L. and Daniel H. Silberberg Associate Professor of Medicine
Director of the Center for Clinical Medical Ethics
Columbia University Vagelos College of Physicians & Surgeons
New York, NY

Notes

1 Jeffrey Bishop, *The Anticipatory Corpse: Medicine, Power, and the Care of the Dying* (Notre Dame: University of Notre Dame Press, 2011), 285.
2 Emmanuel Levinas, *Totality and Infinity: An Essay on Exteriority*, 4th ed. (Dordrecht: Springer, 1991), 50–51.

BIBLIOGRAPHY

'4.3 Nature of Suffering of Those Who Received MAID'. *Second Annual Report on Medical Assistance in Dying in Canada, 2020,* 19–20. Ottawa: Health Canada, 2021. https://www.canada.ca/content/dam/hc-sc/documents/services/medical-assistance-dying/annual-report-2020/annual-report-2020-eng.pdf.

'About Us'. Death with Dignity. https://deathwithdignity.org/about/.

'Quality improvement guidelines for the treatment of acute pain and cancer pain', American Pain Society Quality of Care Committee, *JAMA* 274, no. 23 (1995): 1874–1880.

'Table 1. Characteristics and end-of-life care of 1,905 DWDA patients who have died from ingesting a lethal dose of medication as of January 22, 2021, Oregon, 1998–2020'. Oregon Death with Dignity Act Data Summary (February 2021): 12. https://www.oregon.gov/oha/PH/PROVIDERPARTNERRESOURCES/EVALUATIONRESEARCH/DEATHWITHDIGNITYACT/Documents/year23.pdf.

'Table 2. End of life concerns of participants who died, 2016–2018'. Washington State 2018 Death with Dignity Act Report (July 2019): 11. https://www.doh.wa.gov/Portals/1/Documents/Pubs/422-109-DeathWithDignityAct2018.pdf.

'Ten-Minutes to Midnight' (A Radio Documentary). produced by Alisa Siegel. Prod. edited by Karen Levine. The Sunday Edition, *CBC Radio* (32.27min): 27 October 2019. https://www.cbc.ca/radio/sunday/the-sunday-edition-for-october-27-2019-1.5335017/b-c-man-is-one-of-the-first-canadians-with-dementia-to-die-with-medical-assistance-1.5335025.

Addington-Hall, Julia M. and Saffron Karlsen. 'Age is not the crucial factor in determining how the palliative care needs of people who die from cancer differ from those of people who die from other causes'. *Journal of Palliative Care* 15, no. 4 (1999): 13–19.

Age UK. 'Later life in the United Kingdom 2019'. Fact Sheet. https://www.ageuk.org.uk/globalassets/age-uk/documents/reports-and-publications/later_life_uk_factsheet.pdf.

Ahearn, Laura M. 'Language and agency'. *Annual Review of Anthropology* 30, no. 1 (2001): 109–137.

Aho, James and Kevin Aho. *Body Matters: A Phenomenology of Sickness, Disease, and Illness.* Lanham: Lexington Books, 2009.

Aldwinckle, Russell. *Death in the Secular City.* London: George Allen & Unwin, 1972.

Améry, Jean. *On Ageing: Revolt and Resignation,* translated by John D Barlow. Bloomington: Indiana University Press, 1994.

Andersson, Lars. 'Loneliness research and interventions: A review of the literature'. *Aging and Mental Health 2,* no. 4 (1998): 264–274.

Aronson, Jane. '"I don't want to be a burden": Needing assistance in a context of disentitlement'. *Canadian Woman Studies/Les Cahiers de la Femme* 12, no. 2 (1992): 65–67.

Aronson, Louise. *Elderhood: Redefining Ageing, Transforming Medicine, Reimagining Life.* New York: Bloomsbury, 2021.

Aydede, Mural. 'Preface'. In *Pain: New Essays on Its Nature and the Methodology of Its Study*, edited by M. Aydede, ix–xvii. Cambridge: MIT Press, 2005.

Baars, Jan. *Aging and the Art of Living.* Baltimore: Johns Hopkins University Press, 2012.

Banner, Michael. 'Regarding suffering: On the discovery of the pain of Christ, the politics of compassion, and the contemporary mediation of the woes of the world'. In *The Ethics of Everyday Life: Moral Theology, Social Anthropology, and the Imagination of the Human*, 82–106. Oxford: Oxford University Press, 2016.

———. 'Scripts for Modern Dying: The Death before Death We Have Invented, the Death before Death We Fear and Some Take Too Literally, and the Death before Death Christians Believe In'. *Studies in Christian Ethics* 29, no. 3 (2016): 249–255.

Barbus, Amelia J. 'The Dying Person's Bill of Rights'. *The American Journal of Nursing* 75, no. 1 (1975): 99.

Barth, Karl. *The Church Dogmatics*, translated by Geoffrey Bromiley and Thomas Forsyth Torrance, 14-Volumes. Edinburgh: T&T Clark, 2004.

Barusch, Amanda S. 'The ageing tsunami: Time for a new metaphor?'. *Journal of Gerontological Social Work* 56, no. 3 (2013): 181–184.

Beauchamp, Tom. 'The right to die as the triumph of autonomy'. *Journal of Medicine and Philosophy* 31, no. 6 (2006): 643–654.

Becker, Ernest. *The Denial of Death.* New York: Free Press, 1973.

Beckford, Martin. 'Baroness Warnock: Dementia sufferers may have a duty to die'. *The Telegraph*, 18 September 2008. http://www.telegraph.co.uk/news/uknews/2983652/Baroness-Warnock-Dementia-sufferers-may-have-a-duty-to-die.html.

Bennick, Greg and Patrick Shen (dirs.). *Flight from death: The quest for immortality* (A Documentary Film), narrated by Gabriel Byrne. Arcadia: Transcendental Media, 2003.

Bickenbach, Jerome. 'WHO's definition of health: Philosophical Analysis'. In *Handbook of the Philosophy of Medicine*, edited by Thomas Schramme and Steven Edwards, 961–974. Dordrecht: Springer, 2017.

Bishop, Jeffrey P. *The Anticipatory Corpse: Medicine, Power, and the Care of the Dying.* Notre Dame: University of Notre Dame Press, 2011.

Boffey, Daniel. 'Doctor to face prosecution for breach of euthanasia law'. *The Guardian*, 9 November 2018. https://www.theguardian.com/world/2018/nov/09/doctor-to-face-dutch-prosecution-for-breach-of-euthanasia-law.

———. 'Dutch doctor acquitted in landmark euthanasia case'. *The Guardian*, 11 September 2019. https://www.theguardian.com/world/2019/sep/11/dutch-court-clears-doctor-in-landmark-euthanasia-trial.

Boland, Jason W. and Elaine G. Boland. 'Noisy upper respiratory tract secretions: Pharmacological management'. *BMJ Supportive & Palliative Care* 10, no. 3 (2020): 304–305.

Bonhoeffer, Dietrich. *Creation and Fall: A Theological Exposition of Genesis 1–3*, translated by Douglas Stephen Bax, edited by John W. de Gruchy. Dietrich Bonhoeffer Works, Vol. 3. Minneapolis: Fortress 2004.

———. *Ethics*, translated by Reinhard Krauss, Charles C. West and Douglas W. Stott; edited by Clifford J. Green. Dietrich Bonhoeffer Works, Vol. 6. Minneapolis: Fortress, 2005.

———. *Life Together; Prayerbook of the Bible*, translated by Daniel W. Bloesch and James H. Burtness, edited by Geffrey B. Kelly. Dietrich Bonhoeffer Works, Vol. 5. Minneapolis: Fortress, 1996.

Boztas, Senay. 'Dutch doctor reprimanded for "asking family to hold down euthanasia patient"'. *The Telegraph*, 25 July 2018. https://www.telegraph.co.uk/news/2018/07/25/dutch-doctor-reprimanded-asking-family-hold-euthanasia-patient/

Braider, Christopher. 'Hercules at the Crossroads: Image and soliloquy in Annibale Carracci'. In *Iconoclasm: Turning Toward Pictures*, edited by Ellen Spolsky, 89–116. Lewisburg: Bucknell University Press, 2014.

Bruhn, John and George Henderson. *Values in Health Care: Choices and Conflict*. Springfield: Charles C. Thomas, 1991.

Bueno-Gómez, Noella. 'Conceptualizing suffering and pain'. *Philosophy, Ethics, and Humanities in Medicine* 12, no. 7 (2017): 1–11.

Cacioppe, John T. and William Patrick. *Loneliness: Human Nature and the Need for Social Connection*. New York: W.W. Norton, 2008.

Callahan, Daniel. 'The WHO definition of health'. *The Hastings Center Studies* 1, no. 3 (1973): 77–88.

Carlson, Bryant, Nicola Simopolous, Elizabeth R. Goy, Ann Jackson and Linda Ganzini. 'Oregon hospice chaplains' experiences with patients requesting physician-assisted suicide'. *Journal of Palliative Medicine* 8, no. 6 (2005): 1160–1166.

Case, Anne and Angus Deaton. 'Rising midlife morbidity and mortality, US whites'. *Proceedings of the National Academy of Sciences* 112, no. 49 (2015): 15078–15083.

———. *Deaths of Despair and the Future of Capitalism*. Princeton: Princeton University Press, 2020.

Cassell, Eric J. *The Nature of Suffering and the Goals of Medicine*. Oxford: Oxford University Press, 2004.

Cayley, Cayley. *Ivan Illich: An Intellectual Journey*. University Park: Pennsylvania State University Press, 2021. 443.

Charise, Andrea. '"Let the reader think of the burden": Old age and the crisis of capacity'. *Occasion: Interdisciplinary Studies in the Humanities* 4 (2012): 1–16. https://arcade.stanford.edu/sites/default/files/article_pdfs/OCCASION_v04_Charise_053112_0.pdf.

Chasteen, Alison L. 'The role of age and age-related attitudes in perceptions of elderly individuals'. *Basic and Applied Social Psychology* 22, no. 3 (2000): 147–156.

Chirkov, Valery, Ricahrd M. Ryan, Youngmee Kim and Ulas Kaplan. 'Differentiating autonomy from individualism and independence: A self-determination theory perspective on internalization of cultural orientations and well-being'. *Journal of Personality and Social Psychology* 84, no. 1 (2003): 97–110.

Chrétien, Jean-Louis. 'Body and Touch'. In *The Call and the Response*, 83–131. New York: Fordham University Press, 2008.

Christensen, Kaare, Gabriele Doblhammer, Roland Rau and James W. Vaupel. 'Ageing populations: The challenges ahead'. *Lancet* 374, no. 9696 (2009): 1196–1208.

Cicirelli, Victor G. 'Views of elderly people concerning end-of-life decisions'. *Journal of Applied Gerontology* 17, no. 2 (1998): 186–203.

Cioran, Emil M. *A Short History of Decay*, translated by Richard Howard. London: Penguin, 2018.

———. *On the Heights of Despair*, translated by Ilinca Zarifopol-Johnston. Chicago: University of Chicago Press, 1992.

Commission fédérale de Contrôle et d'Évaluation de l'Euthanasie. 'Communiqué de presse: EUTHANASIE—Chiffres de l'année 2020' [Commission for the Control and Evaluation of Euthanasia. 'Press Release: "EUTHANASIA—Figures for the Year 2020']. https://organesdeconcertation.sante.belgique.be/sites/default/files/documents/cfcee_chiffres-2020_communiquepresse.pdf.

Commission Nationale de Contrôle et d'Évaluation de l'application de la loi du 16 mars 2009 sur l'euthanasie et l'assistance au suicide. 'Cinquième rapport à l'attention de la Chambre des Députés. années 2017 et 2018)' [National Commission for the Control and Evaluation of the Application of the Law of 16 March 2009 on Euthanasia and Assisted Suicide, Fifth report for the attention of the Chamber of Deputies. years 2017 and 2018)]. https://sante.public.lu/fr/publications/r/rapport-loi-euthanasie-2017-2018.html

Copp, Laurel Archer. 'The nature and prevention of suffering'. *Journal of Professional Nursing* 6, no. 5 (1990): 247–249.

Crimmins, Eileen M. 'Trends in the Health of the Elderly'. *Annual Review of Public Health* 25, no. 1 (2004): 79–98.

————— and Hiram Beltrán-Sánchez. 'Mortality and morbidity trends: Is there compression of morbidity?'. *Journal of Gerontology: Social Sciences. Series B, Psychological Sciences and Social Sciences* 66, no. 1 (2011): 75–86.

Critchley, Simon. *Notes on Suicide*. London: Fitzcarraldo Editions, 2017.

Crocker, Louise, L. Clare and K. Evans. 'Giving up or finding a solution? The experience of attempted suicide in later life'. *Aging & Mental Health* 10, no. 6 (2006): 638–647.

de Bellaigue, Christopher. 'Death on demand: Has euthanasia gone too far?'. *The Guardian* (18 January 2019). https://www.theguardian.com/news/2019/jan/18/death-on-demand-has-euthanasia-gone-too-far-netherlands-assisted-dying?CMP=ShareiOS AppOther&fbclid=IwAR3FHnMkBs-cboxgzVOLZ81a8hhYMCEc77e6wT4JuJN8-sQyRdwugUFRe3K4.

Dees, Marianne K., Myrra J. Vernooij-Dassen, Wim J. Dekkers, Kris C. Vissers and Chris van Weel. '"Unbearable suffering": A qualitative study on the perspectives of patients who request assistance in dying'. *Journal of Medical Ethics* 37, no. 12 (2011): 727–734.

de Grey, Aubrey and Michael Rae. *Ending Aging: The Rejuvenation Breakthrough That Could Reverse Human Aging in Our Lifetime*. New York: St. Martin, 2007.

den Hartogh, Govert. 'Suffering and dying well: On the proper aim of palliative care'. *Medicine, Health Care, and Philosophy* 20, no. 3 (2017): 413–424.

Desbiens, Norman A., Nancy Mueller-Rizner, Alfred F. Connors, Jr., Mary Beth Hamel and Neil S. Wenger. 'Pain in the oldest-old during hospitalization and up to one year later. HELP Investigators. Hospitalized Elderly Longitudinal Project'. *Journal of the American Geriatrics Society* 45, no. 10 (1997): 1167–1172.

Dugdale, Lydia S. *The Lost Art of Dying: Reviving Forgotten Wisdom*. New York: HarperOne, 2020.

Duncan, Grant. 'The meanings of "pain" in historical, social, and political context'. *The Monist*, 100, no. 4 (2017): 514–531.

Emanuel, Ezekiel J. 'Why I hope to die at 75'. *The Atlantic* (October 2014). https://www.theatlantic.com/magazine/archive/2014/10/why-i-hope-to-die-at-75/379329/.

Etkind, Marc, ed. *...Or Not to Be: A Collection of Suicide Notes*. New York: Riverhead, 1997.

Eze, Michael Onyebuchi. 'Ubuntu: Toward a new public discourse'. In *Intellectual History in Contemporary South Africa*, 181–192. London: Palgrave MacMillan, 2016.

Fassin, Didier. *Humanitarian Reason: A Moral History of the Present*. Berkeley: University of California Press, 2011.

Fenton, Sarah-Jane. 'Ageing and agency: The contested gerontological landscape of control, security, and independence and the need for ongoing care and support'. *Birmingham Policy Commission* (2014): 1–8. https://www.birmingham.ac.uk/Documents/research/policycommission/healthy-ageing/5-Ageing-and-agency-control-and-independence-updated.pdf.

Fingarette, Herbert and Andrew Hasse. 'A 97-Year-Old Philosopher Faces His Own Death: "What Is the Point?" | The Atlantic'. Online video clip. *The Atlanic*, 18: 12 (14 January 2020). https://www.theatlantic.com/video/index/604840/being-97/.

Fries, James F. 'Aging, natural death, and the compression of morbidity'. *New England Journal of Medicine* 303, no. 3 (1980): 130–135.

Frye, Northrop. *The Educated Imagination*, CBC Massey Lectures. Toronto: House of Anansi, 2002.

Gabriel, Zahava and Ann Bowling. 'Quality of life from the perspectives of older people. *Ageing and Society* 24, no. 5 (2004): 675–691.

Ganzini, Linda, Elizabeth R. Goy and Stephen K. Dobscha. 'Oregonians' reasons for requesting physician aid in dying'. *Archives of Internal Medicine* 169, no. 5 (2009): 489–493.

———, Heidi D. Nelson, Terri A. Schmidt, Dale F. Kraemer, Molly A. Delorit and Melinda A. Lee. 'Physicians' experiences with the Oregon Death with Dignity Act'. *New England Journal of Medicine* 342, no. 8 (2000): 557–563.

———, Stephen K. Dobscha, Ronald T. Heintz and Nancy Press. 'Oregon physicians' perceptions of patients who request assisted suicide and their families'. *Journal of Palliative Medicine* 6, no. 3 (2003): 381–390.

———, Theresa A. Harvath, Ann Jackson, Elizabeth R. Goy, Lois L. Miller and Molly A. Deloril. 'Experiences of Oregon nurses and social workers with hospice patients who requested assistance with suicide'. *New England Journal of Medicine* 347, no. 8 (2002): 582–588.

Giddens, Anthony. *Modernity and Self-Identity: Self and Society in the Late Modern Age*. Cambridge: Polity, 1991.

Gilleard, Chris and Paul Higgs. 'Ageing without agency: Theorizing the fourth age'. *Ageing and Mental Health* 14, no. 2 (2010): 121–128.

——— and Paul Higgs. 'Unacknowledged distinctions: Corporeality versus embodiment in later life'. *Journal of Aging Studies* 45 (2018): 5–10.

Godfrey, Joseph. *A Philosophy of Human Hope*. Dordrecht: Martinus Njhoff, 1987.

Godfrey, Mary, Jean Townsend and Tracy Denby. *Building a Good Life for Older People in Local Communities: The Experience of Ageing in Time and Place*. York: Joseph Rowntree Foundation, 2004.

Goldstein, Kurt. 'Health as value'. In *New Knowledge in Human Values*, edited by Abraham Maslow, 178–188. New York: Harper, 1959.

Gourier, Henry. 'Henri Gourier's Critique in *L'Europe Nouvelle, 20 janvier 1934*'. In *Gabriel Marcel's Perspectives on the Broken World*, edited by Katherine R. Hanley, 153–159. Milwaukee: Marquette University Press, 1998.

Grant, George. 'Thinking about Technology'. In *Collected Works of George Grant*, Vol. 4 (1970–1988), edited by Arthur Davis and Henry Roper, 589–606. Toronto: Toronto University Press, 2009.

Greenhouse, Carol J. *Ethnographies of Neoliberalism*. Philadelphia: University of Pennsylvania Press, 2010.

Gross, Jane. 'Quiet Doctor Finds a Mission in Assisted Suicide Court Case'. *New York Times* (2 January 1997): B1. https://www.nytimes.com/1997/01/02/nyregion/quiet-doctor-finds-a-mission-in-assisted-suicide-court-case.html.

Hagarty, A. Meaghen, Shirley H. Bush, Robert Talarico, Julie Lapenskie and Peter Tanuseputro. 'Severe pain at the end of life: A population-level observational study'. *BMC Palliative Care* 19, no. 60 (2020): doi: 10.1186/s12904-020-00569-2.

Hartog, Iris D., Margot L. Zomers, Ghislaine J. M. W. van Thiel, Carlo Leget, Alfred P. E. Sachs, Cuno S. P. M. Uiterwaal, Vera van den Berg and Els van Wijngaarden. 'Prevalence and characteristics of older adults with a persistent death wish without severe illness: A large cross-sectional survey'. *BMC Geriatrics* 20, no. 342 (2020): doi: 10.1186/s12877-020-01735-0

Hauerwas, Stanley. *The Character of Virtue: Letters to a Godson*. Grand Rapids: Eerdmans, 2018.

Hawkley, Louise C. and John T. Cacioppo. 'Loneliness matters: A theoretical and empirical review of consequences and mechanisms'. *Annals of Behavioral Medicine* 40, no. 2 (2010): 218–227.

Heidegger, Martin. *Parmenides*, translated by André Schuwer and Richard Rojcewicz. Bloomington: Indiana University Press, 1998.

———. *The Question Concerning Technology and Other* Essays, translated by William Lovitt. New York: Harper & Row, 1977.

Hendry, Maggie, Diana Pasterfield, Ruth Lewis, Ben Carter, Daniel Hodgson and Clare Wilkinson. 'Why do we want the right to die? A systematic review of the international literature on the views of patients, carers, and the public on assisted dying'. *Palliative Medicine* 27, no. 1 (2012): 13–26.

Hernandez, Jill Graper. *Gabriel Marcel's Ethics of Hope: Evil, God, and Virtue*. London: Bloomsbury, 2013.

Higgs, Paul and Chris Gilleard. *Rethinking Old Age: Theorising the Fourth Age*. London: Palgrave Macmillan, 2015.

Illich, Ivan. *Limits to Medicine: Medical Nemesis: The Expropriation of Health*. London and New York: Marion Boyars, 1976.

———. *The Right to Useful Unemployment and Its Professional Enemies*. London: Marion Boyars, 1978.

Jaffee, Ina and NPR Staff. 'Silver Tsunami' and other terms that can irk the over-65 set. *Morning Edition* (Radio broadcast). NPR (14 May 2014). https://www.npr.org/2014/05/19/313133555/silver-tsunami-and-other-terms-that-can-irk-the-over-65-set.

Jahn, Danielle R., Kimberley A. Van Orden and Kelly C. Cukrowicz. 'Perceived burdensomeness in older adults and perceptions of burden on spouses and children'. *Clinical Gerontologicst* 36, no. 5 (2013): 451–459.

Jonas, Hans. 'Towards a Philosophy of Technology'. Hastings Center Report (February 1979): 34–43.

Kearney, Richard. 'Carnal hermeneutics'. In *Imagination Now: A Richard Kearney Reader*, edited by M. E. Littlejohn, 99–119. London: Rowman & Littlefield, 2020.

Keefe, Patrick Radden. 'The family that built an empire of pain'. *The New Yorker* (23 October 2017). https://www.newyorker.com/magazine/2017/10/30/the-family-that-built-an-empire-of-pain.

Kemling, Jared. 'Anxiety and fidelity: Gabriel Marcel on existential fear'. *Kinesis* 40, no. 2 (2015): 75–83.

Kingston, Andrew, Louise Robinson, Heather Booth, Martin Knapp, Carol Jagger and MODEM project. 'Projections of multi-morbidity in the older population in England to 2035: Estimates from the Population Ageing and Care Simulation (PACSim) model'. *Age Ageing* 47, no. 3 (2018): 374–380.

Kitchener, Betty and Anthony F. Jorm. 'Conditions required for a law on active voluntary euthanasia: A survey of nurses' opinions in the Australian Capital Territory'. *Journal of Medical Ethics* 25, no. 1 (1999): 25–30.

Knaul, Felicia Marie, Paul E. Farmer, Eric L. Krakauer, Liliana De Lima, Afasan Bhadelia, Xiaoxiao Jiang Kwete, Héctor Arreola-Orelas, et al. 'Alleviating the access abyss in palliative care and pain relief—an imperative of universal health coverage: The Lancet Commission report'. *Lancet* 2017: doi: 10.1016/S0140-6736(17)32513-8.

Kouwenhoven, Pauline S. C., Natasja J. H. Raijmakers, Johannes J. M. van Delden, Judith A.C. Rietjens, Maarte H. N. Schermer, Ghislaine J. M. W. Thiel, et al. 'Opinions of health care professionals and the public after eight years of euthanasia legislation in the Netherlands: A mixed methods approach'. *Palliative Medicine* 27, no. 9 (2013): 273–280.

Kumar, Arun and Nick Allcock. *Pain in Older People: Reflections and Experiences from an Older Person's Perspective*. London: Help the Aged, 2008.

Laslett, Peter. 'The emergence of the third age'. *Ageing and Society* 7, no. 2 (1987): 133–160.

———. *A Fresh Map of Life: The Emergence of the Third Age*. Cambridge: Harvard University Press, 1991.

Levinas, Emmanuel. *Totality and Infinity: An Essay on Exteriority*, 4th edition. Dordrecht: Springer, 1991.

Levy, Becca R. 'Mind matters: Cognitive and physical effects of aging self-stereotypes'. *The Journals of Gerontology: Series B* 58, no. 4 (2003): 203–211.

Linda Ganzini, Elizabeth R. Goy and Stephen K. Dobscha. 'Why Oregon patients request assisted death: Family members' views'. *Journal of General Internal Medicine* 23, no. 2 (2008): 154–157.

Lisowski, R. James. 'Speaking of mystery: Evil and death in the philosophy of Gabriel Marcel and the resulting pastoral applications'. *Marcel Studies* 4, no. 1 (2019): 13–24.

Lloyd-Williams, Mari, Vida Kennedy, Andrew Sixsmith and Judith Sixsmith. 'The end of life: A qualitative study of the perceptions of people over the age of 80 on issues surrounding death and dying'. *Journal of Pain and Symptom Management* 34, no. 1 (2007): 60–66.

Lynch, Scott M. 'Measurement and prediction of aging anxiety'. *Research on Aging* 22, no. 5 (2000): 533–558.

MacKinnon, Donald. 'Death (1955)'. In *Philosophy and the Burden of Theological Honesty: A Donald MacKinnon Reader*, edited by John C McDowell, 307–311. London: T&T Clark, 2011.

———. 'Drama and Memory (1984)'. In *Philosophy and the Burden of Theological Honesty: A Donald MacKinnon Reader*, edited by John C McDowell, 181–188. London: T&T Clark, 2011.

Marcel, Gabriel. 'On the Ontological Mystery'. In *The Philosophy of Existence*, translated by Manya Harari, 5–46. Providence: Cluny, 2018.

———. 'The Broken World: A Four-Act Play'. In *Gabriel Marcel's Perspectives on the Broken World*, edited by Katherine R. Hanley, 31–152. Milwaukee: Marquette University Press, 1998.

————. 'The concept of spiritual heritage'. *Confluence: An International Forum* 2, no. 3 (1953): 3–15.

————. *Being and Having*: An Existentialist Diary, translated by Katherine Farrer. Westminster: Dacre, 1949.

————. *Creative Fidelity*, translated by Robert Rosthal. New York: Fordham University Press, 2002.

————. *Homo Viator: Introduction to a Metaphysic of Hope*, translated by Emma Craufurd and Paul Seaton. South Bend: St Augustine's, 2010.

————. *Man against Mass Society*, translated by G. S. Fraser. South Bend: St Augustine's, 2008.

————. *Metaphysical Journal*, translated by Bernard Wall. London: Rockliffe, 1952.

————. *The Mystery of Being, Volume I: Reflection and Mystery*, translated by G. S. Fraser. South Bend: St Augustine's, 2001.

————. *The Mystery of Being, Volume II: Faith and Reality*. South Bend: St Augustine's, 2001.

Marcuse, Herbert. *One Dimensional Man: Studies in the Ideology of Advanced Industrial Society*. Boston: Beacon, 1991.

McGreal, Chris. 'US medical group that pushed doctors to prescribe painkillers forced to close'. *The Guardian* (25 May 2019). https://www.theguardian.com/us-news/2019/may/25/american-pain-society-doctors-painkillers.

McKee, Kevin and Marynn Gott. 'Shame and the ageing body'. In *Body Shame: Conceptualization, Research, and Treatment*, edited by P. Gilbert and J. Miles, 75–89. London: Routledge, 2002.

McKenny, Gerald P. *To Relieve the Human Condition: Bioethics, Technology, and the Body*. Albany: State University of New York Press, 1997.

McMaughan, Darcy, Rachel Edwards and Bita Kash. 'The Methusian catastrophe'. *Primary Health Care* 3, no. 2 (2013): 1–3.

McPherson, Christine J., Keith G. Wilson and Mary Ann Murray. 'Feeling like a burden: Exploring the perspectives of patients at the end of life'. *Social Science & Medicine* 64, no. 2 (2007): 417–427.

Meghani, Salimah, Eeeseung Byun and Rollin M Gallagher. 'Time to take stock: A meta-analysis and systematic review of analgesic treatment disparities for pain in the United States'. *Pain Medicine* 13, no. 2 (2012): 150–174.

Mende-Siedlecki, Peter, Jennie Qu-Lee, Robert Backer and Jay J. Van Bavel. 'Perceptual contributions to racial bias in pain recognition'. *Journal of Experimental Psychology. General* 148, no. 5 (2019): 863–889.

Messer, Neil. *Flourishing: Health, Disease, and Bioethics in Theological Perspective*. Grand Rapids: Eerdmans, 2013.

Mester, Philip. 'Gabriel Marcel: Mystery of Being'. *Dominicana* 48, no. 2 (1963): 129–136.

Mesthene, Emmanuel G. 'Technology and Wisdom'. In Technology and Social Change, edited by Emmanuel G. Mesthene, 57–62. Indianapolis: Bobbs-Merrill, 1967.

————. *Technological Change: Its Impact on Man and Society*. New York: New American Library, 1970.

Monforte-Royo, Cristina, Christian Vallavicencio-Chávez, Joachin Tomás-Sábado, Vinita Mahtani-Chugani and Albert Balaguer. 'What lies behind the wish to hasten death? A systematic review and meta-ethnography from the perspective of patients'. *PLoS ONE* 7, no. 5 (2012): e371117 (1–16).

Montanari, Franco, Chr. Tsagalis and Antonios Rengakos, eds. *Brill's Companion to Hesiod*. Leiden: Brill, 2009.

Morgan, David. 'Pain: The unrelieved condition of modernity'. *European Journal of Social Theory* 5, no. 3 (2002): 307–322.

Morris, David. *The Culture of Pain*. Berkeley: The University of California Press, 1993.

Morris, John N., Samy Suissa, Sylvia Sherwood, Susan M. Wright and David Greer. 'Last days: A study of the quality of life of terminally ill cancer patients. *Journal of Chronic Diseases* 39, no. 1 (1986): 47–62.

Morris, Steven. '"Right thing to do": Guernsey begins assisted dying debate'. *The Guardian*, 16 May 2018. https://www.theguardian.com/society/2018/may/16/right-thing-to-do-guernsey-begins-assisted-dying-debate.

Mortimer, Ian. 'The triumph of the doctors: Medical assistance to the dying, C. (1570–1720. The Alexander Prize Essay)'. *Transactions of the Royal Historical Society* 15 (2005): 97–116.

Moyse, Ashley John. 'Responsibility for the broken body: Exploring the invitation to respond to the presence of the other'. In *Treating the Body in Medicine and Religion: Jewish, Christian, and Islamic Perspectives*, edited by John J. Fitzgerald and Ashley John Moyse, 17–28. London: Routledge, 2019.

———. *Reading Karl Barth, Interrupting Moral Technique, Transforming Biomedical Ethics*. New York: Palgrave, 2015.

———. *The Art of Living for the Technological Age: Towards a Humanizing Performance*. Minneapolis: Fortress, 2021.

Nia Williams, Charlotte Dunford, Alice Knowles and James Warner. 'Public attitudes to life-sustaining treatments and euthanasia in dementia'. *International Journal of Geriatric Psychiatry* 22, no. 12 (2007): 1229–1234.

Nietzsche, Friedreich. *The Will to Power*, translated by Walter Kaufmann and Reginald J. Hollingdale. New York: Vintage, 1968.

———. *Thus Spoke Zarathustra*, translated by Adrian Del Caro. Cambridge: Cambridge University Press, 2006.

———. *Human, All Too Human: A Book for Free Spirits*, translated by Helen Zimmern. Edinburgh: T.N. Foulis.

O'Callaghan, Paul. 'Hope and Freedom in Gabriel Marcel and Ernst Bloch'. *The Irish Theological Quarterly* 55, no. 3 (1989): 215–239.

O'Mahony, Seamus. 'The compression of morbidity: A real phenomenon or just wishful thinking?', *The Value of Death* (19 September 2019). https://commissiononthevalueofdeath.wordpress.com/2019/09/19/the-compression-of-morbidity-a-real-phenomenon-or-just-wishful-thinking/.

———. 'Medical Nemesis 40 years on: The enduring legacy of Ivan Illich'. *The Journal of the Royal College of Physicians of Edinburgh* 46, no. 2 (2016): 134–139.

———. *Can Medicine Be Cured: The Corruption of a Profession*. London: Head of Zeus, 2019.

———. *The Ministry of Bodies*. London: Head of Zeus, 2021.

———. *The Way We Die Now*. London: Head of Zeus, 2016.

Ovid. *Metamorphoses*, translated by Anthony S Kline. http://ovid.lib.virginia.edu/trans/Ovhome.htm.

Palenčár, Marián. 'Gabriel Marcel and the question of human dignity'. *Human Affairs* 27, no. 2 (2017): 116–130.

Paul, John II. *Salvifici Doloris*. Apostolic Letters. Rome, 11 February, 1984. http://www.vatican.va/content/john-paul-ii/en/apost_letters/1984/documents/hf_jp-ii_apl_11021984_salvifici-doloris.html.

Paz, Octavio. 'Este Lado'. In *Árbol adentro*, 33. Barcelona: Seix Barral, 1987.

Pearlman, Robert A., Clarissa Hsu, Helene Starks, Anthony L. Back, Judith R. Gordon, Ashok J. Bharucha, Barbara A. Koenig and Margaret P. Battin. 'Motivations for physician-assisted suicide: Patient and family voices'. *Journal of Gerontology and Internal Medicine*, 20, no. 3 (2005): 234–239.

Pérez, Julia Urabayen. 'El humanismo trágico de Gabriel Marcel: el ser humano en un mundo roto'. *Estudios de Filosofía*, 41 (2010): 35–59.

Pestinger, Martina, Stephanie Stiel, Frank Elsner, Guy Widdershoven, Raymond Voltz, Friedemann Nauck and Lukas Radbruch. 'The desire to hasten death: Using grounded theory for a better understanding "when perception of time tends to be a slippery slope" '. *Palliative Medicine* 29, no. 8 (2015): 711–719.

Plath, Debbie. 'Independence in old age: The route to social exclusion?'. *British Journal of Social Work* 38, no. 7 (2008): 1353–1369.

———. 'International policy perspectives on Independence in old age'. *Journal of Aging & Social Policy* 21, no. 2 (2009): 209–223.

Portacolone, Elena. 'The myth of independence for older Americans living alone in the Bay Area of San Francisco: A critical reflection'. *Ageing and Society* 31, no. 5 (2011): 803–828.

Quill, Timothy E. 'Death and Dignity'. *New England Journal of Medicine* 324, no. 10 (1991): 691–694.

———, Sally Norton, Mindy Shah, Yvonne Lam, Charlotte Fridd and Marsha Buckley. 'What is most important for you to achieve? An analysis of patient responses when receiving palliative care consultation'. *Journal of Palliative Medicine* 9, no. 2 (2006): 382–388.

Randall, Albert. *The Mystery of Hope in the Philosophy of Gabriel Marcel*. Lewiston: Edwin Mellon, 1992.

Regionale Toetsingscommissies Euthanasie. 'Jaarverslag 2017' – 'Jaarverslag 2020'. April 2018, 2019, 2020, 2021.

Reuter, Kevin and Justin Sytsma. 'Unfelt pain'. *Synthese* 197, no. 4 (2020): 1777–1801.

Ridenour, Autumn Alcott. 'Suffering, death, and the significance of presence'. In *Treating the Body in Medicine and Religion: Jewish, Christian, and Islamic Perspectives*, edited by John J. Fitzgerald and Ashley John Moyse, 184–196. London: Routledge, 2019.

Ritzer, George. *The McDonaldization of Society in the Digital Age*, 9th edition. Los Angeles: Sage, 2018.

———. *The McDonaldization of Society: An Investigation into the Changing Character of Contemporary Life*. Thousand Oaks: Pine Forge, 1993.

Robinson, David S. '*Peccatorum Communio*: Intercession in Bonhoeffer's Use of Hegel'. *Studies in Christian Ethics* 28, no. 1 (2015): 86–100.

Robinson, Fiona. 'Resisting hierarchies through relationality in the ethics of care'. *International Journal of Care and Caring* 4, no. 1 (2020): 11–23.

Rodgers, Beth L. and Kathleen V. Cowles. 'A conceptual foundation of human suffering in nursing care and research'. *Journal of Advanced Nursing* 25, no. 5 (1997): 1048–1053.

Romaioli, Diego and Alberta Contarello. 'Redefining agency in late life: The concept of "disponibility" '. *Ageing and Society* 39, no. 1 (2019): 194–216.

Ron, Pnina. 'Elderly people's attitudes and perceptions of aging and old age: The role of cognitive dissonance'. *Geriatric Psychiatry* 22, no. 7 (2007): 656–622.

Rosa, Hartmut. *Social Acceleration: A New Theory of Modernity*, translated by Jonathan Trejo-Mathys. New York: Columbia University Press, 2013.

————. *Resonance: A Sociology of Our Relationship to the World*, translated by James C. Wagner. Cambridge: Polity, 2019.

————. *The Uncontrollability of the World*, translated by James C. Wagner. Cambridge: Polity, 2021.

Rose, Gillian. *Love's Work: A Reckoning with Life*. New York: New York Review, 1995.

Rowe, John W. and Robert L. Kahn. *Successful Aging*. New York: Pantheon, 1998.

Rubinstein, Robert L. and Kate de Medeiros. 'Successful Aging'. gerontological theory and neoliberalism: A qualitative critique'. *The Gerontologist* 55, no. 1 (2015): 43–42.

Rurup, Mette L., Bregje D. Onwuteaka-Philipsen, H. Roeline W. Pasman, Miel W. Ribbe and Gerrit van der Wal. 'Attitudes of physicians, nurses and relatives towards end-of-life decisions concerning nursing home patients with dementia'. *Patient Education and Counseling* 61, no. 3 (2006): 372–380.

Szalavitz, Maia. 'Opioids feel like live. That's why they're deadly in tough times'. *The New York Times* (6 December 2021). https://www.nytimes.com/2021/12/06/opinion/us-opioid-crisis.html.

Schoeni, Robert F., Vicki A. Freedman and Linda G. Martin. 'Why is late-life disability declining?'. *Milbank Quarterly* 86, no. 1 (2008): 48–89.

Schopenhauer, Arthur. 'Additional remarks on the doctrine of the suffering of the world '. In *Parerga and Paralipomena: Short Philosophical Essays*, Vol. 2, translated/edited by Adrian del Caro and Christopher Janaway, 262–275. Cambridge: Cambridge University Press, 2015.

Second Annual Report on Medical Assistance in Dying in Canada, 2020. Ottawa: Health Canada, 2021. 17.

Selzer, Richard. *The Exact Location of the Soul: New and Selected Essays*. New York: Picador, 2001.

Shaw, Rhonda and Matthew Langman. 'Perceptions of being old and the ageing process'. *Ageing International* 42, no. 1 (2017): 115–135.

Sin, Chih Hoong. 'Older people from white-British and Asian-Indian backgrounds and their expectations for support from their children'. *Quality in Ageing and Older Adults* 8, no. 1 (2007): 31–41.

Slegers, Rosa. 'Reflections on a Broken World: Gabriel Marcel and William James on Despair, Hope and Desire'. In *Hope against Hope: Philosophies, Cultures and Politics of Possibility and Doubt*, edited by Janet Horrigan and Ed Witse, 55–74. Leiden: Brill, 2010.

Sleight, Vivian. 'Hope and despair'. *Journal of the Royal Society of Medicine* 97, no. 7 (2004): 354.

Smadar, Bustan. 'A scientific and philosophical analysis of meanings of pain in studies of pain and suffering'. In *Meanings of Pain*, edited by Simon van Rysewyk, 107–128. Cham: Springer International, 2016.

Smith, Alexander K., Irena Stijacic Cenzer, Sara J. Knight, Kathleen A. Puntillo, Eric Widera, Brie A. Williams, W. John Boscardin and Kenneth E. Covinsky. 'The epidemiology of pain during the last 2 years of life'. *Annals of Internal Medicine* 153, no. 9 (2010): 563–569.

Smith, Cecil. 'Vase with representation of Herakles and Geras'. *The Journal of Hellenic Studies* 4 (1883): 96–110.

Sørensen, Anders Dræby. 'The paradox of modern suffering'. *Tidsskrift for Forskning i Sygdom og Samfund*, 7, no. 13 (2010): 131–159.

Spaemann, Robert. 'In defense of anthropomorphism'. In *A Robert Spaemann Reader: Philosophical Essays on Nature, God, & the Human Person*, translated/edited by D. C. Schindler and Jeanne Heffernan Schindler, 77–96. Oxford: Oxford University Press, 2015.

Stark, James. *The Cult of Youth: Anti-ageing in Modern Britain*. Cambridge: Cambridge University Press, 2020.

Stenner, Paul, Tara McFarquhar and Ann Bowling. 'Older people and "active ageing": subjective aspects of ageing actively'. *Journal of Health Psychology* 16, no. 3 (2011): 467–477.

Stoneking, Carole Bailey. 'Receiving Communion: Euthanasia, Suicide, and Letting Die'. In *The Blackwell Companion to Christian Ethics*, edited by Stanley Hauerwas and Samuel Wells, 375–387. Malden: Blackwell, 2006.

Strauss, Claudia. 'The imaginary'. *Anthropological Theory* 6, no. 3 (2006): 322–344.

Stringfellow, William. 'The Moral Reality Named Death'. In *An Ethic for Christians and Other Aliens in a Strange Land*, 67–94. Eugene: Wipf & Stock, 2004.

Sullivan, M. J. L., Heather Adams, Sharon Horan, Denise Maher, Dan Boland and Richard Gross. 'The role of perceived injustice in the experience of chronic pain and disability: Scale development and validation'. *Journal of Occupational Rehabilitation* 18, no. 3 (2008): 249–261.

———. Whitney Scott and Zina Trost. 'Perceived injustice: A risk factor for problematic pain outcomes'. *Clinical Journal of Pain* 28, no. 6 (2012): 484–488.

Suzman, Richard M., David P. Willis and Kenneth Manton, eds. *The Oldest Old*. Oxford: Oxford University Press, 1992.

Sweeney, Terence. 'Against Ideology: Gabriel Marcel's Philosophy of Vocation'. *Logos* 16, no. 4 (2013): 179–181.

Szasz, Thomas S. *Pain and Pleasure*. New York: Basic Books, 1957.

Tauber, Alfred I. *Confessions of a Medicine Man: An Essay in Popular Philosophy*. Cambridge: MIT Press, 2002.

Taylor, Charles. *A Secular Age*. Cambridge: Belknap, 2007.

———. 'Modern social imaginaries'. *Public Culture* 14, no. 1 (2002): 91–124.

———. *Modern Social Imaginaries*. Durham: Duke University Press, 2003.

Tester, Susan, Gill Hubbard, Murna Downs, Charlotte MacDonald and John Murphy. 'Frailty and institutional life'. In *Growing Older. Quality of Life in Old Age*, edited by Alan Walker and Catherin Hagan Hennessy, 209–224. Maidenhead: Open University Press, 2004.

Thorpe, Deborah Moorehead. 'Comprehensive pain care: The relief of pain and suffering'. *Dimensions in Oncology Nursing* 4, no. 1 (1990): 27–29.

Torres, Sandra and Gubhild Hammerström. 'Speaking of 'limitations' while trying to disregard them: A qualitative study of how diminished everyday competence and aging can be regarded'. *Journal of Aging Studies* 20, no. 4 (2006): 291–302.

Tutu, Desmond. *No Future without Forgiveness*. London: Rider, 1999.

van Esch, Harriëtte J., Martine E. Lokker, Judith Rietjens, Lia van Zuylen, Carin C. D. van der Rijt and Agnes van der Heide. 'Understanding relatives' experience of death rattle'. *BMC Pyschology* 8, no. 62 (2020): doi: 10.1186/s40359-020-00431-3.

van Holsteyn, Joop and Margo Trappenburg. 'Citizens' opinions on new forms of euthanasia: A report from the Netherlands'. *Patient Education and Counseling* 35, no. 1 (1998): 63–73.

van Humbeeck, Liesbeth, Let Dillen, Ruth Piers, Nele van den Noortgate. 'Tiredness of life in older persons: A qualitative study on nurses' experiences of being confronted with this growing phenomenon'. *The Gerontologist* 60, no. 4 (2019): 735–744.

van Wijngaarden, Els J., Carlo J W Leget and Anne Goossensen. 'Till death do us part: The lived experience of an elderly couple who chose to end their lives by spousal self-euthanasia'. *The Gerontologist* 56, no. 6 (2016): 1062–1071.

———, Carlo Leget and Anne Goossensen. 'Experiences and motivations underlying wishes to die in older people who are tired of living: A research area in its infancy'. *OMEGA—Journal of Death and Dying* 69, no. 2 (2014): 191–216.

———, Els, Carlo Leget and Anne Goossensen. 'Reading to give up on life: The lived experience of elderly people who feel life is completed and no longer worth living'. *Social Science and Medicine* 138 (2015): 257–264.

VanderWeele, Tyler J. 'Suffering and response: Directions in empirical research'. *Social Science and Medicine* 224 (2019): 58–66.

Vrancken, Mariet A. E. 'School of thought on pain'. *Social Science and Medicine* 29, no. 3 (1989): 434–444.

Walker, Alan. 'The economic "burden" of ageing and the prospect of intergenerational conflict'. *Ageing & Society* 10, no. 4 (1990): 377–396.

Wand, Anne P. F., Carelle Peisah, Brian Draper and Henry Brodaty. 'Why do the very old self-harm? A qualitative study'. *American Journal of Geriatric Psychiatry* 26, no. 8 (2018): 862–871.

Warnes, Anthony M. 'Being old, old people and the burdens of burden'. *Ageing and Society* 13, no. 3 (1993): 297–338.

Warraich, Haider. *Modern Death: How Medicine Changed the End of Life*. London: Duckworth Overlook, 2017.

Waters, Brent. 'Technology, distractions, and the care of the body'. *Human Flourishing Blog*. October 2019. https://www.patheos.com/blogs/humanflourishing/2019/10/technology-distractions-and-the-care-of-the-body/.

WHO. *Constitution*, Geneva: World Health Organization, 1948. https://www.who.int/about/governance/constitution.

WHO. *International classification of functioning, disability and health*, Geneva: World Health Organization, 2001. https://www.who.int/standards/classifications/international-classification-of-functioning-disability-and-health.

Wilkinson, Iain. *Suffering: A Sociological Introduction*. Cambridge: Polity, 2005.

Willcutt, Zachary. 'Marcel and Augustine on immortality: The nothingness of the self and the exteriorization of love as the way to eternity'. *Marcel Studies* 5, no. 1 (2020): 1–18.

Williams, David A. and Beverly E. Thorn. 'An empirical assessment of pain beliefs'. *Pain* 36, no. 3 (1989): 351–158.

Wright, Stephen. 'When dignity'. *Nursing Standard* 19, no. 33 (2005): 30–31.

Yu, Cheng-Ling. 'Hope and despair: A discussion on the atheistic existentialist, evolutionary biologistic and intersubjective accounts of hope'. *Marcel Studies* 5, no. 1 (2020): 19–36.

Zee, Art Van. 'The promotion and marketing of oxycontin: Commercial triumph, public health tragedy'. *American Journal of Public Health* 99, no. 2 (2009): 221–227.

INDEX